First-Time Mom

Understanding Hypnobirthing Methods and Prepare Yourself for pregnancy. Learn the New Way to Calm Crying and Help Your Newborn Baby Sleep Longer

Katharine Marie

of any of the information provided by this book. This disclaimer applies to any loss, damages or injury caused by the use and application, whether directly or indirectly, of any advice or information presented, whether for breach of contract, tort, negligence, personal injury, criminal intent, or under any other cause of action.

You agree to accept all risks of using the information presented inside this book.

You agree that by continuing to read this book, where appropriate and/or necessary, you shall consult a professional (including but not limited to your doctor, attorney, or financial advisor or such other advisor as needed) before using any of the suggested remedies, techniques, or information in this book.

Table of Contents
Hypnobirthing

Baby Sleep Training

Hypnobirthing

Hypnosis and Mindfulness Techniques for a Calm and Pain Free Birth. Prepare Yourself for Pregnancy and Childbirth, Be a Perfect First-Time and Mindful Mom for grow a confident newborn

Katharine Marie

Introduction

Hypnobirthing is a strategy for torment the executives that can be utilized during work and birth. It includes utilizing a blend of representation, unwinding and profound breathing methods. Breathing practices have for quite some time been a piece of antenatal classes. Hypnobirthing takes this and includes unwinding, representation and care systems to assist you with focusing on your body and the introduction of your child. Hypnobirthing can be utilized with every other sort of relief from discomfort and be added to your introduction to the world arrangement.

What are the strategies and systems utilized in hypnobirthing?

Controlled relaxing

Breathing profoundly, in through your nose and out through your mouth, can assist you with staying quiet and diminish inconvenience in labor.

Representation

Representation is the place you envision the introduction of your child and what you need to occur. It very well may be something extremely explicit or increasingly broad, similar to an inclination you need to have. For instance, you could picture what it will feel like to hold your infant skin to skin after they've been conceived. It resembles a practice in your psyche to assist you with feeling increasingly arranged and positive.

'I simply continued breathing and concentrated on anything I could discover, which wound up being a perfect wool!'

Reflection may assist you with focusing on your body and child during work, while overlooking any additional clamor or things going on around you. 'My significant other made me an unwinding collection to use all through work and pregnancy. It truly helped me to discover quiet quietness in the clinical medical clinic condition.'

Does hypnobirthing work?

For the present, there is restricted investigation into hypnobirthing. A randomized investigation of 680 ladies financed by the NHS in 2013 didn't decisively show that it was compelling. This implies it will work for certain ladies and not others. Here are a portion of the reasons that you may decide to take a stab at hypnobirthing:

Hypnobirthing can assist you with overseeing pressure hormones, for example, adrenalin, and lessen tension, which should prompt a more quiet birth. During work, your body creates a concoction called oxytocin, which helps progress your work. Stress hormones influence the creation of oxytocin, and make your work longer.

Overseeing pressure may likewise diminish a portion of the dread and agony experienced during work.

Now and again, hypnobirthing has been appeared to make work shorter.

Working on hypnobirthing – regardless of whether it's at a class, with a book or CD – may assist you with feeling progressively arranged and in control when work begins. It might assist you with adapting to nerves in the event that you had a past awful birth understanding. Hypnobirthing may lessen the requirement for medications and therapeutic intercession. Be that as it may, you can have extra relief from discomfort also on the off chance that you need to. It very well may be added to any birth plan and the strategies can be utilized any place you conceive an offspring – in a medical clinic or birth focus, or at home.

Hypnobirthing may profit you after birth as well, with some proof indicating that it can bring down the opportunity of postnatal wretchedness.

'I discovered helping my accomplice conceive an offspring utilizing hypnobirthing exceptionally fulfilling. Learning the procedures together implied I had the option to talk her through the influx of every compression, reminding her to remain engaged and loose and that she was responsible for the experience. It had so a lot of effect having the option to accomplish something positive during her work and to see her dealing with the torment herself.' Nigel. Peruse progressively about his experience...

Are there weaknesses to hypnobirthing?

Working on hypnobirthing doesn't mean sudden things won't occur. A birth free from medicinal intercessions or inconveniences can never be ensured. In any case, figuring out how to unwind and remain quiet may assist you with feeling more in charge during work if things don't go to design.

'We read a book and tuned in to sound contemplation tapes yet they didn't fill in as we truly didn't submit whenever to it.' Daisy

Most hypnobirthing classes and regimens are run secretly, so all things considered, you should pay.

Chapter 1

What Is Hypnobirthing?

Hypnobirthing, as defined by dictinary.com, is an approach of managing pain, as well as stress and anxiety, throughout childbirth. This includes various therapeutic relaxation techniques, such as deep breathing and visualization.

It's essentially taking those old beliefs and thoughts around childbirth, which were triggering anxiety, and then transforming those old beliefs to new ones that will positively equipping you for childbirth. Hypnobirthing then includes adding functional healing techniques and teaching you to change your attitude to give you the favorable birthing experience that you prefer.

It is a birthing strategy that consolidates extensive breathing, unwinding, representation, self-mesmerizing and direction for both you and also your birthing partner. You can use the systems in labor as well as transportation to aid you in adapting to pain.

Some people may be put off by the word 'hypnobirthing'. If you know nothing about hypnobirthing, the word may conjure up images of stage hypnosis where people are hypnotised to eat onions as if they were apples, swirly patterns, mind control and goodness knows what else! This is thanks to stage hypnosis shown on some television programmes, which is done for entertainment purposes only.

We all enter the state of hypnosis several times a day, so it is a very familiar, natural state to our minds and bodies and we can all do it. Ever relaxed watching a film and become totally engrossed in it, so that you don't notice someone speaking to you? Or started reading a novel and before you know it you have lost contact with time - time has flown by in what felt like a short space of time? How about when you've been driving a familiar route and suddenly you arrive at your destination but you don't really remember parts of the journey? These are all examples of naturally occurring trans states or hypnosis, but in the example of driving a car you would immediately switch into a conscious state and avoid danger if a car pulled out in front of you!

To de-mystify it, hypnobirthing is a simple antenatal preparation for birth that involves:

self-hypnosis;

easy to learn techniques to work with your breath;

guided relaxations;

an understanding about the power of the mind and the mind-body connection;

developing an understanding about the powerful effect of language on the mind and body during labour;

positive affirmations;

using visualisation;

understanding the power of hormones released during natural labour and the birth environment during labour;

informed decision making and an understanding of your options and choices during labour and birth;

learning how to release fears;

learning about how the body works during labour and birth and what factors can help or hinders this process (some of these factors we have already covered in previous chapters).

So, hypnobirthing is a complete antenatal education and preparation in and of itself, combined with some very practical elements. It might be useful to think of it as a mindset-reset or overhaul.

An essential part of a hypnobirthing course (and indeed any good antenatal course or preparation for birth book) is the process where you learn practical skills to use to enable you to remain calm and relaxed during your labour and birth, combined with knowledge and informed decision making to enable your birth to be a positive experience.

Women who practice hypnobirthing frequently report that they are able to relax and enjoy their pregnancy and feel more positive preparing for labour and birth. They enjoy listening to the guided relaxations, fall asleep listening to the MP3s and learn to trust their bodies. Women already know how to give birth, but sadly, it is common that faith and trust in the process has been lost along the way. Hypnobirthing gives women and their birth partners a set of tools and techniques that can help them to use their already present, natural birthing instincts.

The specific practice of breathing techniques and changed mindset can often result in a more comfortable birthing experience, with couples reporting that they felt calmer and in control, however their birth unfolded. Hypnobirthing has become very popular, with many women using the techniques and some midwives and maternity units offering classes.

Hypnobirthing is not necessarily about removing pain, but rather, it is about reframing it and understanding how your body is working to birth your baby. The breathing and mindset practices help to allow you to let go, give yourself over to your body rather than fighting against or resisting the surges, which reduces or eliminates fear and panic, with all the problems that they bring.

Whilst some women report that they only experienced tightenings or pressure during their labour, other women report that they did feel pain, but that they did not feel out of control or frightened by it. They understood what its purpose was, that it is their surges working hard to bring their baby to them rather than something wrong happening.

 If you decide to undertake a hypnobirthing course, it is best to start earlier in the pregnancy rather than later, with most couples starting between 20-

30 weeks of pregnancy. This is to enable lots of repetition in order to embrace a different mindset around birth. However if you come to hypnobirthing later than 30 weeks, it is important not to be put off – you will just need to commit yourself and intensify your practice, rather than building it up slowly.

Advantages of hypnobirthing

Hypnobirthing techniques help a woman to relax, which in turn:

Means that she is going to be breathing deeply and calmly, which increases oxygen to herself and her baby.

Means she will be activating the parasympathetic response of 'calm and connection' ensuring the uterus, placenta and baby will have a good blood supply.

Surges are likely to be more efficient.

The 'fight or flight' mechanism is not stimulated.

Endorphin production, the body's natural and super powerful painkiller, is enhanced.

Women and partners feel empowered.

Birth partners are very much involved and have an important role.

It is common that no medication is needed.

Women are informed and understand how their body works in labour.

Women report feeling calm and in control, whatever turn their birth takes.

There are no harmful side effects to the mother or baby – in fact babies benefit from the increased oxygen from the calm, regular, deep breathing.

Practising hypnobirthing during pregnancy will often mean that the woman is able to feel more positive approaching the labour and birth. She will have a tool kit to enable her to deal with challenges or 'wobbly' moments, which means that she is able to enjoy her pregnancy without unnecessary fears hanging over her.

Parents often report they enjoy a little time out a few times a week to focus on the pregnancy, baby and each other.

A woman can also practice alone and falling asleep to the MP3s is fine.

Potential disadvantages of hypnobirthing:

Consistent time and effort is required in order to get the full benefits of hypnobirthing – but this is often described as relaxing, enjoyable and positive, so is this really a disadvantage?

Doing a hypnobirthing course costs money, but many women successfully can practice hypnobirthing by reading books and listening to the relaxation MP3s.

You may not have a practitioner in your area – but a Skype class or online course may be an option.

Sometimes women feel it didn't work for them, or that it only helped them for part of their labour and feel disappointed about this.

What is hypnosis?

Many people think hypnosis is a mysterious thing that someone does to them. They may picture a person lying on a couch, with the hypnotherapist beside them working their

magic while the patient is passive. In actual fact, all hypnosis is self-hypnosis and during hypnosis no one can make you do anything you do not want to do and you will only accept suggestions that are morally right for you.

The mind is of course incredibly complex, but try thinking of it as existing in two parts: the conscious and subconscious mind. The conscious mind is where we spend most of our time, but it's actually the weakest part of the mind. It regulates decision-making, processing of information, perception through the five senses, critical thinking, analytical thinking, spacial awareness, judgements, awareness of self and awareness of time.

The subconscious is the most powerful part of the mind. It regulates memory, imagination, dreaming and instinct, and it relays information back to the conscious. It is also our permanent memory, so everything we've ever experienced is stored here, like huge database. As we go through life, this database of information develops into our beliefs and habits, making us who we are today. Our beliefs dictate how we think and the actions we will take.

Roughly speaking, when a person becomes relaxed in hypnosis they are in an enhanced state of awareness, concentrating on the words being said. In this state the judging, analytical conscious mind is suppressed allowing access to the powerful subconscious mind.

The hypnobirthing scripts your partner reads out to you and/or the MP3s you listen are then able to suggest positive ideas and concepts directly to your subconscious around trusting your body's ability to birth your baby - and these seeds of positivity become firmly planted in the subconscious. As the subconscious mind is a more powerful and instinctive force than the conscious mind, this is the part which has to change in order to amend old, negative beliefs.

The subconscious mind, which does not distinguish between what is real and what is imaginary, is open to all sorts of positive realities, such as 'you are prepared and ready to relax into a wonderful birth experience'.

A person must be willing and interested, as only they can allow themselves to lie down, begin deep breathing, to relax and listen to the guided relaxations. No one can make them use their imagination to visualise certain events.

It is good that hypnosis is voluntary, as this means that you are always completely in control of yourself, but it does also mean a person needs to genuinely be interested in giving hypnobirthing a go and making a commitment to using the power of the mind. Hypnobirthing would be useless if you had no interest or belief in it.

So yes, you are still aware of what is going on around you, but you are open to positive suggestions and less focussed on your immediate surroundings.

To use hypnobirthing requires you to practice the techniques. Most of us have grown up thinking of labour and birth as something that we have to 'get through', and that it will be incredibly painful and frightening. We've heard our auntie's, our mother's and our friends' birth stories, not to mention how birth is portrayed in the media and on TV shows, and so unless you're very fortunate, it's usually pretty negative stories.

To unlearn these unhelpful programmes, stories and beliefs we have about birth takes time and repetition and setting aside a little time in your week to focus on this. When actions and ideas are repeated over and over they become habits and beliefs which can be very powerful.

Self-hypnosis is one way to clear that out and fill that section with positivity instead. Then, when you go into labour, your mind will access the positive birth information you've shelved in your subconscious. Your brain will believe that 'birth is OK and safe', which can prevent the fear-pain-cycle and raised adrenalin levels negatively affecting your natural release of helpful birth hormones.

When a labouring woman is relaxed, her surges can do the job they are meant to do. This means that her uterine muscles work together as nature intended – the upper segment of the uterus contracts strongly and with each successive contraction the muscle fibres of the upper segment become shorter and thicker (retraction) which in turn draws the weaker, thinner part of the lower uterus up and in doing so this dilates the cervix, gradually moving the baby downwards. With each contraction the upper part of the uterus becomes thicker and thicker. Tension in the mind and body causes the cervix to remain taut and closed, meaning that the two sets of muscles work against each other, which results in an increased experience of pain and a slower labour.

Chapter 2

The Hypnobirthing Philosophy

The "hormonal physiology of childbearing" here alludes to propagation related biologic procedures from pregnancy through the baby blues and infant periods in connection to inborn, endogenous hormone frameworks. "Physiologic childbearing" alludes to childbearing complying with sound biologic forms. Predictable and cognizant proof finds that physiologic childbearing encourages advantageous (salutogenic) results in ladies and children by advancing fetal preparation for birth and wellbeing during work, improving work viability, furnishing physiologic help with work pressure and torment, advancing maternal and infant advances and maternal adjustments, and streamlining breastfeeding and maternal-newborn child connection, among numerous procedures.

The perinatal period is profoundly touchy for mother and child in connection to hormonal and other biologic procedures. Practices that advance (through ideal strategies and framework limits), support (with direct encouraging practices), and secure (from aggravation) physiologic childbearing may have intensified, continuous advantages—for instance, through supporting breastfeeding.

Contemporary childbearing has profited by numerous medicinal advances, and from profoundly gifted and submitted maternity care suppliers, particularly for moms and infants who require extraordinary care. Be that as it may, current high paces of maternity care intercessions might be disadvantageous for the solid dominant part. Basic maternity care practices and mediations can affect the hormonal physiology of mother and infant, as indicated by physiologic understandings and human and creature ponders. Effects on hormonal physiology and ramifications for mother or potentially infant may happen in the perinatal period or past. For instance, prelabor cesareans are related with decreased fetal/infant epinephrine-norepinephrine because of loss of the "catecholamine flood," which may add to expanded respiratory and different morbidities. Longer-term impacts from perinatal hormonal interruptions are conceivable in ladies and infants, as per temporary human discoveries and strong creature inquire about.

Center hormonal physiology subjects and standards repeat all through outcomes orchestrated in this report, uncovering significant interconnections at numerous levels and after some time, as pursues.

Maternal and newborn child endurance during childbirth is clearly basic for conceptive achievement, yet similarly significant for long haul endurance are fruitful lactation and maternal–baby connection promptly following birth. These hormonally-intervened forms are entwined and nonstop with the biologic procedures of parturition. Disturbance of perinatal hormonal physiology may in this way sway work and birth, yet in addition breastfeeding and maternal–baby connection. As people share numerous conceptive procedures with different vertebrates, creature explore enlightens human hormonal physiology, particularly where human research is right now restricted.

Hormonal physiology is interrelated, facilitated, and commonly controlled among mother and infant to enhance results for both. For instance, maternal and fetal status for work is unequivocally adjusted at the physiologic beginning of term work to streamline work proficiency and maternal and infant changes. Also, skin-to-skin contact after birth commonly directs maternal and infant oxytocin frameworks. As a general guideline, consequences for maternal hormonal physiology sway fetal/infant hormonal physiology, and the other way around.

From pregnancy through work and birth, breastfeeding, and maternal–baby connection, hormonal procedures of physiologic childbearing envision and get ready for forthcoming procedures and organic needs. For instance, prelabor upregulation of maternal uterine oxytocin receptors advances work proficiency, and prelabor epinephrine-norepinephrine receptor upregulation advances fetal adjustments to work hypoxia and infant changes through the fetal catecholamine flood.

The hormone frameworks depicted here have complex collaborations in the perinatal period, including advancing or hindering each other's action. This can intensify hormonal impacts, prompting the pinnacles that portray physiologic birth. For instance, late-work oxytocin tops, advanced by significant levels of prolactin and oxytocin itself, help with the pushing stage. So also, over the top pressure and stress hormones may upset work progress by means of hormonal interorchestration.

Hormonal disturbances can be intensified when one mediation requires and prompts another that is utilized to screen, avoid, or treat its symptoms. This

17

acceleration of innovation can additionally disturb hormonal physiology and present additional dangers for mother and infant. For instance, the decrease in maternal oxytocin that for the most part pursues organization of epidural absense of pain may prompt utilization of engineered oxytocin to redress. Drawn out utilization of engineered oxytocin may desensitize the oxytocin receptor framework and increment the danger of baby blues drain.

Non-physiologic exposures during the touchy perinatal period may upset posterity hormone frameworks, with enhanced and additionally suffering natural, formative, as well as conduct impacts, as found in creature posterity, likely by means of epigenetic programming impacts. High-caliber, long haul human thinks about after fetal/infant presentation to perinatal medications and intercessions are exceptionally restricted. In this way, the present proof based way to deal with recognizing protected and compelling consideration, in light of present moment development and constrained assessment of hormonally-interceded results, for example, breastfeeding, may not give sufficient shields to moms and children. Essentially, ordinary shorter-term pharmacologic contemplations of fetal/infant medicate presentation (e.g., portion, span, digestion) may not sufficiently protect the infant. Ebb and flow levels of vulnerability about long haul impacts propose look into needs and backing keeping away from unneeded mediations.

The physiologic (unconstrained) beginning of term work is a complex and not entirely got procedure. Basic for endurance, its planning is believed to be basically controlled by the infant's development, by means of fetal cortisol generation, facilitated with the mother's preparation for parturition, through estrogen creation and different forms. Timing of the physiologic beginning of term work is hard to anticipate because of typical variety in the length of human development.

With the physiologic beginning of work at term, maternal and fetal frameworks are completely prepared and absolutely adjusted for sheltered, viable, work and birth, and for ideal baby blues physiologic advances, including breastfeeding inception and maternal–infant connection, as indicated by physiologic understandings, and human and creature thinks about. Physiologic prelabor arrangements happen in the weeks, days, and (in creature considers) hours before the beginning of work.

Hypnosis' Rule in Hypnobirthing

The hypnobirthing manuscripts your companion reads out to you and/or the MP3s you listen to are able to recommend positive concepts and ideas directly to your subconscious around trusting your body's capability to birth your infant - as well as these seeds of positivity become strongly grown in the subconscious. As the subconscious mind is a much more powerful and instinctive force than the conscious mind, this is the part that has to transform in order to amend old, unfavorable ideas.

The subconscious mind, which does not distinguish between what is real and what is imaginary, is open to all types of positive facts, such as "you are ready and all set to relax into a wonderful birth experience."

Each step of any type of hypnotherapy is completely volunteer. A person must want to relax, as only they can enable themselves to rest, to begin deep breathing, and to pay attention to the led relaxations. No one can make them utilize their imagination to visualize particular events.

Pregnant mothers, when using hypnobirthing are in total control of themselves. Hypnobirthing would be worthless to someone who had no rate of interest or idea in it.

Some individuals state, after they have actually utilized self-hypnosis or saw a hypnotherapist, "It can't have worked as I was aware of what was taking place around me throughout the session. I listened to the phone ring and individuals speaking outdoors". Nonetheless, self-hypnosis merely means having quiet, undisturbed time, focusing inwardly, or on a certain topic, and also enabling yourself to drift into a deeply relaxed state of mind - by hearing your companion read out among the scripts in this book in a positive and repeated means.

So yes, you are still aware of what is going on around you, but you are open to positive tips as well as less concentrated on your immediate environments.

Chapter 3

Inner Preparation Of Childbirth And Beyond

IT'S THE second class of the MBCP course, and tonight we will learn a bit more about each other and go deeper into mindfulness practice. Once everyone has settled comfortably, I begin.

"I'd like to invite each of you to join me in a little guided reflection. Allow your eyes to close if you feel comfortable doing so, and come to the sensations of breathing. Taking a moment now, imagine yourself standing beside a well. Perhaps it's a well you've seen before, or one that you imagine right now. Notice the landscape around this well, the weather, the temperature of the air. Looking at the ground by your feet, pick up a stone. Feel its weight, its texture against the skin of the palm of your hand. Now, holding the stone over the opening of the well, let it become a question.

The classroom is silent. After a time I ring the bells and everyone opens their eyes. Through the sharing that follows, we come to a better understanding of who each of us is and what has brought us to this moment in this room. Benefiting from seeing each other in an expanded context, we can now do the same with our mindfulness practice.

Transition is the phase of delivery where your cervix is fully dilated to 10 cm and the baby is positioned to move down through the birthing canal. At this phase, your contractions will be at their most intense and you will have the urge to push. Coordinating your pushing with your contractions will give you the best results. There are several positions that can be used for the delivery of your baby. You and your birthing team will pick the one that works best for you and your delivery

Delivery Positions

The position you use to deliver your baby is very important. Some positions actually speed up the delivery of your baby by using gravity to help push the baby down and out and maximizing the work that your body is doing with each contraction and push. Other positions can actually slow down the delivery process.

Many women think of lying in the hospital bed, feet in stirrups and knees akimbo when they imagine delivering their baby. There are several reasons for this. First, it is the scene that we see played out in the movies and on television most of the time. Secondly, for years this is the preferred position of hospitals as it gives the doctors and nurses the most control and easiest access. However, this is actually one of the least effective positions for delivery. Lying down in bed physically limits your hips' ability to expand by a full thirty percent. This position works against gravity rather than with it. It increases the risk of needing the aid of forceps or a vacuum to get the baby out. It also greatly increases your risk of perineum tearing. In this section, we will explore some other delivery positions that actually aid your body in the delivery process.

- Kneeling/leaning- Kneeling beside the bed and leaning forward or bending over a birthing ball are very good positions for delivering your baby. This position is particularly good for keeping your contractions strong and allowing you to rock back and forth as you bear down into the contraction. It also utilizes the force of gravity in moving your baby down and out. This position also allows your birthing partner greater access to support you by putting their arms around you during contractions, holding your hands and keeping your hair out of your face. Those little things mean so much during delivery.

- On all fours- This is a great position if you are experiencing back labor. Though this position can somewhat slow contractions, it minimizes the risk of tearing the perineum. It is one of the best positions for delivering large babies.

- Sitting- Sitting is a good alternative position if you must stay in bed for medical reasons. It makes better use of gravity than lying down but you are sitting on your tailbone which can make it harder for the baby to come down.

- Lying down- This position actually works against gravity so it can slow down labor. In some cases, they need to slow down labor if the baby is coming too fast before full dilation has occurred. This is also a good position if the mother is completely worn out. She can rest between contractions easier. It is also the best position if there are medical concerns that the doctors and nurses need to be able to address quickly as it gives them the best access.

It is important that you are psychologically and physically comfortable with the position that you chose to deliver your baby in. Every position has pros and cons. There is no right or wrong choice. There is only the right choice for you in this delivery.

Pushing

Once your cervix is fully dilated, you will begin to feel the urge to bear down and push. Your contractions may have more time between them once again, allowing you to have a moment to rest in between contractions and pushing. The urge to push feels a lot like the feeling you get when you need to empty your bowels. You may actually have a bm while pushing. This is perfectly natural and nothing to be ashamed of. This is nature's way of making sure that nothing is obstructing the birth canal.

There is something very primal and empowering about birthing your baby. Many women feel very connected to their own bodies and their baby during this phase of delivery. Some women even describe that time seems to stand still during this phase and they enter into a world of their own. This feeling makes the time spent pushing seem shorter as they are so focused on their babies and their own bodies.

If you are in one of the upright positions, the force of gravity itself is aiding in the birthing of your baby. This adds to the primal and connected feeling that this phase of delivery brings. Follow your body's instincts and push when it tells you to push. This will speed up delivery and minimize the risk of tearing.

Your breathing is very important to this stage of delivery. Breathe deep into your abdomen, this delivers the most oxygen to your muscles and also helps to focus you through the pain. Once your baby's head crowns your doctor or midwife will ask you to stop pushing for a moment while they make sure that the umbilical cord is positioned correctly. During this time use the 'blowing out a candle' technique to resist the urge to push.

This phase of delivery ends with the healthy delivery of your baby! Congratulations!

After the delivery of your baby, you will deliver the placenta. This is relatively painless. Most women are so focused on their new baby that this barely registers. The nurse or midwife may push on your abdomen to help deliver the placenta or they may give you a shot of Pitocin in your leg to speed the process along. Once the placenta is delivered the doctor or midwife will examine it to be sure the entire placenta was delivered intact. It is important that they get all of the placenta delivered to avoid infection later on.

Postnatal Baby Care

Having skin to skin contact with your baby is a very important part of the initial bonding experience. Both mother and father should bond with their baby using this method. Having skin to skin contact with their parents has been proven to have other physical benefits as well. Babies who get skin to skin contact with their parents have better heart and lung function compared to babies who do not have the same skin to skin contact. They also have better glucose and heat regulation, cry less, both mother and infant are proven to rest better and nursing is an easier transition for both baby and mom.

Here are some tips for skin to skin contact with your baby.

- Hold your baby to your chest directly after birth. If there is a medical reason that mom can not do this, dad can put the baby on his chest. Hold your baby and let them get used to the smell of your skin, the sound of your breathing and the sound of your voice.

- Keep your baby in your room as much as possible. Some hospitals try to give mom a break by taking the baby to the nursery. This can interfere with the bonding experience. Keep your baby in the room with you, when at all possible.

- Become a baby wearer.- There are many different baby carrier options from different kinds of slings to seated carriers. Find a sling-style that works for you and wear your baby. This will free up your hands to do the things that you need to do and provide your baby the comfort and closeness that they need. Babywearing also makes nursing easier.

- Talk and sing to your baby while wearing them and feeding them. This provides great comfort to your baby, creates deep bonding and has been proven to improve nursing.

- Give your baby tummy time. By placing your baby on their stomach you are helping to strengthen their neck muscles as they start lifting their head. Tummy time doesn't have to be on the floor. You can have tummy time with your baby laying on your stomach, skin to skin. This will encourage them to lift their head to look at you and will continue your bonding. Just be sure to keep one hand on their back for safety.

- Infant massage- There is growing evidence that infant massage is calming for babies but also has great physical benefits. Slowly and gently rub each part of your baby's body. Watch them to make sure that you are not rubbing too hard. It is best to wait 45 minutes after feeding to do this because massaging to soon after feeding can cause them to spit up their milk.

- Father and baby skin to skin time.- It is important that daddy and baby have skin to skin time to bond. It will give the baby a sense of security and they will learn their father's voice, smell, touch, and breathing. Be sure to include daddy in skin to skin time.

Chapter 4

Nutrition

Food is my medicine, my medicine my food"

Preparing for the birth means preparing yourself mentally, emotionally, and physically. You must look after yourself in order to be able to look after your unborn baby. The first step to doing this is to look at your diet.

These days pregnant women are well informed of the importance of a healthy diet during pregnancy. Not only does good nutrition help your baby to develop, it also has a huge impact on your health.

It helps your body to perform physically, mentally, and emotionally. A healthy, balanced diet helps you to stay fit and strong and the nutrients your food provides affects your hormone balance thus playing a part in how you think and feel about things.

Based on my research and experience below is an overview of the most important nutritional advice as i understand it for a healthy pregnancy.

The ayurvedic way

According to the ayurvedic system, every person is born with a constitution which is identified under 3 categories (vata, pitta and kapha). So this means that depending on your constitution you should eat foods accordingly. If you google an ayurvedic test to see if you are vata, kapha or pitta you will be able to see what type you come under.

If you still don't know go and find a practicing ayurvedic doctor and they will tell you. There are super foods which one person can eat which would be poison to another so why not find out what suits your particular type.

There is a fantastic book which is written by ayurvedic doctor andreas moritz called **timeless secrets of health and rejuvenation** which contains a fantastic test for anyone who wants to find out their constitution.

This book is a bible of health tips for anyone who wants good health. Trust me you will be happy you invested in this amazing book. Ayurvedic medicine has been around for over 5000 years and contains a lot knowledge for living a healthy life.

Vegetarian or vegan pregnancy

There is a huge misconception out there surrounding a vegetarian diet and iron. My iron levels were perfect all the way through my pregnancy, much to the surprise of everyone.

By eating a vegetarian diet you are also ensuring less toxins enter you and the baby. If energy is everything then think about taking the energy of dead meat into your body. This animal, more than likely, died in fear for its life and so the meat carries the energy of fear. What happens when we eat it? Of course we then take on this fear.

There are two basic human emotions - fear and love - and all emotions can come under these two categories be it anger, hate, sorrow or whatever. So if there is only fear and love we want to accentuate the feelings of love and positive higher vibrations especially in our pregnancy.

If we can stay in a state of love and in positive higher vibrations we are of course more likely to feel confident and self-assured, and in turn have a confident birth. There are many ways to raise our vibrations to that of love and away from fear. Eating a plant based diet is a great place to start.

A further note on meat and protein; once an animal dies, the oxygen supply is cut off and so cells begin to break down causing the meat to start to decay and turn colour and become purified protein. This coupled with the process of cooking and preserving the meat causes the protein to coagulate and the human body cannot use coagulated protein for cell- building.

This is why meat is very toxic to the body and is treated as a pathogen by the intestines, which in turn stimulates an intense immune response. Note: you may feel a boost in energy from this immune response which you may interpret as good. But over a long time the body only gets weaker and weaker from eating meat and indeed ages prematurely.

If we were meant to eat meat then we would have the teeth to tear and grind meat and the digestive juices to digest it. I will not detail here the immense suffering and cruelty of the meat industry and the fact that it is causing so much damage to our environment. The truly sad part is that the meat industry actually causes starvation because this industry is using so much of the grain and land which could be feeding the people of the planet.

Protein

The truth is babies do not need much protein at all and in fact human breast milk only contains a trace of protein. There is a common belief that meat makes you strong and healthy but when you consider animals with great strength such as an elephant, a horse or a rhinoceros, who are completely vegetarian, you can see that this is an absolute lie.

When it comes to fish you are also dealing with coagulated protein which your body cannot use. In terms of toxins such as heavy metals and chemicals, fish puts every pregnant woman and her developing fetus at risk. When you consider that populations who eat the most meat have the shortest life expectancy, and the highest level of disease such as the rising epidemics of heart disease and cancer, we can see that the rise in meat consumption is a major cause for this explosion.

Another point worth making, regarding the consumption of meat (particularly while pregnant), is the fact that the colon has a direct influence on the reproductive system. It is extremely important that in pregnancy the bowel functions regularly and is kept clean.

Meat is so indigestible and tends to make us constipated. Dry foods such bread, potatoes, pastas, and popcorn should also be avoided. We should try and introduce unrefined fats and oils such as the amazing coconut oil. I add 2 or 3 tablespoons into my porridge in the morning and it tastes really nice.

Start with a smaller amount as it has great laxative powers. The growing baby needs plenty of fats as do all pregnant women.

It is very safe to have enemas, colemas and colonics in pregnancy and in fact it was custom for every pregnant woman to receive an enema before birth in years gone by. Keep hydrated by eating food with high water content and of course drink good quality water at room temperature (never cold).

Cow's milk

Avoid cow's milk. Although it is rich in calcium, this calcium is not absorbable for us humans and it actually leeches calcium out of our bones. A powerful source of calcium is the humble sesame seed which contains a massive 1160 milligrams of calcium per 100 grams. The super-grain, chia seed, is packed with numerous minerals too. Remember to check your constitution or body type first to see if these foods suit your particular type because a super food for one person can be bad for another.

Virgin coconut oil

Virgin coconut oil is proven to be an antiviral and antibacterial agent due to the high levels of lauric acid. Lauric acid is also found in mother's milk. This is one of the reasons coconut milk is an excellent alternative when breast milk is not available.

This amazing oil keeps the colon super clean, which is so important particularly when you are pregnant. Coconut oil keeps the body alkaline;

and because of its anti-parasitic and anti-yeast properties, it naturally prevents yeast infections in women.

In populations who consume coconut oil, such as areas in the tropics, it has been shown that digestion issues are rare. Issues like heart disease, colitis, colon cancer, haemorrhoids and ulcers were also very uncommon.

Coconut oil also removes toxins and has been found to promote weight loss and keep muscles lean. Coconut oil keeps hypothyroidism balanced. This oil is the safest of all the oils and perfect for cooking with, as it does not oxidize with heat.

Start with small amounts as it is quite a powerful laxative. Eventually you can take up to 3 ½ tablespoons every day. I just add 3 tablespoons in my porridge in the morning and it tastes lovely.

Tip 1: this oil makes a terrific moisturizer for the skin too!

Tip 2: coconut oil is packed with nutrition so why not add a spoon of it to your porridge in the morning. A word of caution here; as coconut oil is a strong laxative, start slowly and begin with one teaspoon. Then build up to a tablespoon or two over a few weeks as your body gets used to it.

Iodine

Iodine is an essential mineral for a healthy pregnancy, and for women's health in particular. It is a vitally important nutrient that has an impact on every organ and system in the body. It is particularly important for regulating the thyroid gland.

The thyroid releases hormones into the bloodstream affecting almost every part of the body, including the brain. These hormones are crucial for the development of your unborn baby, in particular - brain function. When the thyroid becomes under active this is known as hypothyroidism.

A major cause of hypothyroidism is a lack of iodine in the body. For the first 12 weeks of pregnancy, before the unborn baby's thyroid becomes active, the mother is the sole source of thyroid hormones. When the mother is lacking in iodine, her and her foetus are hypothyroid. This increases the risk of the baby developing mental retardation.

It is also interesting that canadian thyroid expert dr. David derry spent years treating his patients with unusually high doses of iodine for various thyroid conditions. He had a particular interest in the relationship between iodine and breast cancer and wrote a book called **breast cancer and iodine: how to prevent and how to survive breast cancer**.

It is always better that we try to get all our nutrients from our food but sometimes it is necessary to take supplements in order to meet our recommended daily intake. The guidelines for pregnant women are about 220 micro grams (mg) per day, and for breastfeeding women about 290 mg per day. The following is a list of foods that are naturally rich in iodine and should be used as a rough guide only because the amount of iodine can vary in most foods:

One gram of dried seaweed/sea vegetable like wakame = 80 mg

Himalayan pink salt and celtic grey salt = 77 mg

One baked potato including the skin = 60mg

Half a cup of cooked navy beans = 32 mg

One cup of strawberries = 13 mg

If you feel you are not getting enough iodine through your diet, you could take iodine supplements. Nascent iodine is the most hypo-allergenic form of supplemental iodine, or if you are robust, lugol's solution is a popular and inexpensive form. 2 drops of 5% lugol's solution contains around 6 mg of iodine.

Make sure you are not allergic to lugol's solution – rub a drop into the inside of your arm and leave for 24 hours. If there is no reaction it is safe to use.

For internal doses take lugol's solution in 4-6 oz of water or orange juice. Best taken with food and early in the day.

Red raspberry leaf (rubus idaeus)

I'm sure you are familiar with the popular juicy red raspberry fruit. Not only is this delicious little fruit packed with nutrients, the leaf of its plant has been used for centuries for its medicinal properties. The raspberry leaf has many benefits and is very often used for pregnancy related conditions, such as morning sickness and bleeding gums. It is a rich source of magnesium, iron and calcium. It also contains vitamins e, b1, and b3.

Many women take raspberry leaf tea during pregnancy, particularly because they believe it helps to tone the muscles of the uterus, making contractions easier and assisting with the delivery of the baby and placenta. It is also used to help stimulate the production of breast milk, regulate the menstrual cycle, decreasing heavy blood flow and painful menstrual cramps.

Raspberry leaf tea is a popular way to take this herb but it is also available in the form of capsules, tinctures and tablets.

As with all medicines, including herbal medicines, there are precautions you must take if you decide you want to take raspberry leaf.

Because it is a mild uterine stimulant, it is advisable to avoid raspberry leaf during the first trimester.

Begin with one cup a day and build up to three cups.

If you experience strong uterine cramps (known as braxton hicks contractions) stop taking it.

If you have a history of premature labour, miscarriage, multiple birth or any other complications, it may be wise for you to avoid raspberry leaf.

Do inform your midwife that you are considering taking it.

Here is a short list of foods i like to include in my diet for their nutritional values:

Almonds (for their calcium) are a delicious healthy food that you can eat on their own as a snack or add to salads and other dishes such as rice, noodles and couscous. It is best to soak almonds either overnight in cool water or briefly in boiling water to remove skins which are indigestible. Please avoid drinking cow's milk as it is better suited to a big suckling calf like nature intended. Recipe for almond milk here:

Almond milk

To make almond milk, soak one and a half cup of almonds overnight, remove the water and you are left with nice enlarged almonds. Now you can either put boiling water on the almonds and remove the skins, or you may want to wait and strain the skins off later. I prefer to remove skins immediately. It just takes a couple of minutes.

After about 4 minutes in boiling water the skins should simply slip off easily. Simply add 3 cups of water and blend.

You can add a few dates, honey, vanilla or cinnamon at this stage to get a lovely sweet flavour. I like to combine honey and vanilla to my almond milk. Once the milk is lovely and frothy your almond milk is ready and can be kept in the refrigerator for up to 3 days. If you prefer cashew nuts then use the same method and make yourself some nutritious cashew milk instead. (p.s. Cashews are full of magnesium).

Note: if you want to leave the skins on you may use a muslin cloth to strain the skins after blending

Marine phytoplankton

Possibly the most nutritional food on the planet. 10 -15 drops of this stuff will go a long way in making sure you and your baby are getting all the vitamins and minerals you require at this important time.

I would strongly recommend you start taking this supplement before you are pregnant to ensure you are in perfect health for your expectant pregnancy.

Marine phytoplankton is a trusted source of folate (folic acid), not to mention life sustaining high grade nutrients such as niacin, riboflavin, thiamine, omega 3 essential fatty acids (epa and dha), protein, chlorophyll, amino acids, vitamins, and trace elements. It contains various minerals, including selenium, iron, iodine and magnesium.

Marine phytoplankton is for this reason referred to as the king of super foods.

All the scientific research indicates that marine phytoplankton may be the most important food on planet earth.

Many women experience low iron levels in pregnancy and by simply taking marine phytoplankton this would safely bring their iron levels back not to mention all the other benefits of this amazing health food.

Magnesium oil

This mineral is a godsend in pregnancy. Magnesium is referred to as the relaxing mineral.

The easiest way to absorb magnesium oil is through the skin. You can buy a bottle and just spray it on, every other day. Spray on any area which is aching. I use the ancient minerals brand.

As epsom salts are a form of magnesium, you can take regular epsom salt baths. Dissolve the salts for 15 minutes in hot water before getting into the bath and soak in the bath for 20 minutes.

You can also consume magnesium rich foods such as dark leafy greens, avocado, nuts, seeds and beans. A large amount of our population is deficient in magnesium and is completely unaware of it.

Chapter 5

The Power Of Mind

Your mind has two parts—the aware and the unaware (additionally referred to as the conscious and subconscious). If we were to compare your mind to an iceberg, the peak would be the logical, aware part of our mind, the part that claims, "I ought to slim down" or "I should be more careful not to lose control". The majority listed below the surface area would be your subconscious mind, where 90% of your thinking power originates from.

The Subconscious Mind

Your subconscious mind controls all things that occur automatically, for instance, your breathing, digestion, your routines, and any thoughts or feelings that show up outside your control.

The goal of your subconscious mind is to maintain your health and security. It filters millions of items of information that are sent from your senses to your brain, and it uses this information to decide if there are any risks close by. It then either automatically moves you away from danger or pain or towards satisfaction.

It can do this successfully due to the fact that it doesn't spend time "thinking" on things (that is your conscious mind's job). It merely responds.

Our memories, beliefs, values, and previous choices develop part of this filtering process. Our unconscious mind utilizes these four things to help us to become aware of the most essential pieces of detail in our environment.

Sometimes, however, if fear dominates us, the unconscious mind may incorrectly believe that the fear is something we desire since it's something that we are frequently considering. This is why, sometimes, our fears will come to light—our emotional mind is frequently functioning to make our ideas a fact. If we think of something enough, our unconscious mind thinks that it is because we desire it.

Several issues can be credited to our unconscious mind acting upon inaccurate, obsolete, or insufficient information. As an example, an idea you had as a child might still serve as the source of heartache in adulthood.

The issue is that as soon as we have created an idea about something, this influences the way our mind filters the information we take in, so we, then, tend to focus on things that confirm that idea.

There is a maxim known as Orr's Law. It says, "What the thinker thinks, the prover will prove." Therefore, a child constantly told that they would never amount to anything that may begin to believe this. For, in the eyes of a child, the grown-up must be right. Their unconscious mind holds the belief that "I am no good" and their mind begins to filter all of their experiences through this belief to confirm it—"I told you I can't do anything right. I did it wrong again..."

Due to this, their self-esteem and self-confidence drops. Then, their belief becomes self-fulfilling as they keep acting in a manner that verifies that belief, even into adulthood.

The Link Between Mind and Body

Just as the beliefs that you hold can cause you discomfort, distress, or hurt, they can also help to bring you success.

Whatever your belief about yourself or something else happens to be, that is what you will act upon. Sometimes you don't even know why. This also suggests that you cannot act upon something that you do not, at least to some degree, believe in. According to this theory, if you don't believe it, your subconscious mind will filter it out of your conscious mind.

Every home convenience that we have, from peanut butter to microwaves was invented by somebody who believed they could do it. Without believing that it is possible, there can be no action taken.

It took Thomas Edison 800 tries to get the light bulb to work right. Can you picture what the world today if he had stopped believing it possible? Or if he had believed himself a failure after his 799th try? You produce your future, likewise, through the power of your beliefs.

Fortunately, you have the capability to transform your beliefs. Think back. There have been numerous points in your life when you held beliefs about yourself that you no longer do. Typical instances consist of Santa Claus, the Easter Bunny, and the Tooth Fairy.

Overcoming faulty beliefs about yourself or about life is possible, regardless of who you are or how old you are. It begins with a mindset.

The Thoughts, Feelings, Behavior Cycle

Your mindset (what you believe and think), the way you feel, and your behavior are all linked, and changing any of them will affect the others.

However, the mindset—the beliefs and thoughts, typically come first. Even if it's a subconscious thought, remember that it still influences your feelings, as well as your behavior. And our thoughts typically relate to the circumstance we're in at the time.

Recognizing your state of mind, by looking at what you think, will permit you to analyze whether it is assisting you to get to the success you desire or preventing you by bringing you unhappiness.

However, if you can take control of your thoughts, then you can consequently take control of your life. This is a lot simpler than merely trying to "quit" worrying. It's nearly impossible to just quit something when the belief that has caused the feeling in the first place is still present and working its "magic".

I'm sure that you have heard the saying, "Seeing is believing". I am suggesting to you that the opposite is true. You must have faith in what you truly desire or want before it will come to pass.

If you don't believe that something will go well, it probably won't. That's why when things go against what we assume will happen, we say, "Well!

That was surprising!" Remember, "What the thinker thinks, the prover will prove."

Talking negatively can become a self-fulfilling prophecy. The uncertainty negative speaking—"I can't", "I won't", "I don't know", etc., cause tension, concern, or worry, and it stops you from getting what you really desire.

So exactly how can you end up having the labor and delivery that you want?

It's simple, really! Take control by letting go of anxiety, and swap this with self-confidence!

Worry and Fear

We must learn to let go of fear. But before we can, we must first understand a little bit about fear and the fact that our mind sometimes holds to fear, thinking it is helping us.

Apprehension, worry, anxiety, concern, nervousness, and panic are frequently manifestations of fear. They are psychological responses to something that appears harmful or something that a person is scared of.

These feelings can be healthy and balanced if they keep us safe from threats. They can work as a warning, telling us to be cautious, but sometimes this fear triggers more distress than is necessary. This is because we are usually fearful of what could occur - not just what is occurring.

When we are fearful or sense a threat, our mind causes the stress action in our bodies by sending signals that cause physical reactions, including an increased heart rate and high blood pressure, muscular tissue tension, rapid breathing, and enhanced sensitivity. Our muscles tense to ensure that our body can respond by fighting against the danger of running away from the things that we are afraid of - this is known as the "fight or flight disorder". Primarily, blood is moved far from non-essential muscle mass and body organs to those muscles that may need it for fighting or running away.

The fight or flight response continues until the mind decides that the risk has passed. Nevertheless, your muscle mass can only stay on "red alert" for so long. So, if you stay fearful, your muscles will eventually tire out and quit working properly. So, in giving birth, people often tend to experience discomfort merely due to fear or being tense or because they are anticipating that giving birth to hurt.

Just like any other emotion, fear can be mild, moderate, or extreme. This depends upon the person and the way their mind works. And, believe it or not, close to 80% of pregnant women approach labor with some degree of fear. The issue with fear is that it prevents two abilities that are vital to successful labor and delivery: relaxation and concentration.

Chapter 6

Mindfulness In Everyday Life

When the time comes for labor and birth, you will have the knowledge, pain practice, and communication skills to drop into the present moment and work with the birthing process, however it unfolds. And once the baby has been born, informal practice may predominate, at least for a time. Your new mindfulness teacher— the small one coming soon— is going to keep you pretty busy with informal practice. Nursing and feeding and burping and diaper changing, bathing and playing, comforting and rocking and attuning to cues— these are the informal mindfulness practices of parenting, and why informal practice is such great preparation, not only for childbirth but for parenting as well.

So how do you start your informal practice? In the beginning you just pick one or two activities in your daily life and fully commit to being there as you engage in them: brushing your teeth, making morning coffee or tea, driving to work, greeting a co-worker, turning on the computer, answering the telephone, chopping vegetables, or washing the dishes after dinner. These moments all become part of your informal mindfulness practice, which of course are the very real moments of your life as you live it.

Listed here are a few general guidelines for being more awake and aware in your daily life.

1. Whenever possible, do just one thing. Then do the next. Then the next. Mindfully, that is.

Part of the incredible stress of modern life has to do with how much we think we need to get done every day. The result is that we can find ourselves completely absorbed in doing almost all the time. Multitasking becomes the order of the day. However, when we begin to practice paying attention to one thing at a time, fully, and then the next and then the next, we may find that we are less stressed. Paradoxically, we may also find that the quality of whatever we are engaged in improves and that we actually accomplish more, with greater joy.

In truth, there is no such thing as multitasking. Research shows that the brain can pay attention to only one thing at a time. We can move our attention swiftly back and forth from one task to the next, which gives us the illusion that we're doing more than one thing, but we're not; we're serial processing extremely quickly. When we push ourselves to multitask, we're asking our brain to do something it wasn't really designed to do. We can do it, but it takes a huge amount of energy— and we are certainly asking ourselves to do more than we can do well. The result? We feel frustrated, irritable, overwhelmed, confused,and exhausted. In a word, stressed.

These days technology, as wonderful as it is, has added a huge burden of complexity to our daily lives, so much so that scientists are investigating what we are doing to our brains with all the hours we spend online, texting, tweeting, e-chatting, and Skyping. Yet one thing hasn't changed: our children still need our undivided attention, an increasingly difficult thing to get in an overly stimulating world. This is why it's so important to make part of our preparation for parenting the practice, whenever possible, of consciously paying attention to just one thing at a time.

2. Throughout your day, whenever you can remember, bring your attention to your breath.

As we learned in Chapter 6, when we feel anxious, frightened, angry, hurried, or worried, our stress hormones do their fight-or-flight thing and our body changes; breathing rate increases, as does our heart rate and our blood pressure. When we feel at ease and relaxed, we are reregulating back into balance with calm and connection; breathing, heart rate, and blood pressure all decrease. When you can remember to come back to the breath throughout your day, you get a reading on your inner landscape; coming back to the sensations of breathing, you are intentionally helping to calm and rebalance your body and mind. The Three-Minute Breathing Space can be a wonderful practice to enfold into your everyday life.

3. Practice bringing awareness to your moment-to-moment bodily sensations (touching, hearing, seeing, smelling, tasting), as well as your thoughts and emotions, while you are engaged in everyday life. Bringing mindfulness into your daily activities means doing whatever you are doing and knowing that you are doing it. Physical sensations, thoughts, and emotions are all doorways to awareness and the present moment.

4. Practice Being with Baby. As you learned in Chapter 4, let the sensations from the baby's movements call you back into the present moment

throughout your day. If circumstances permit, pause from whatever you are doing and bring your full attention directly to the sensations the baby is creating inside your body— the quick little pokes, the rolling movements, the rhythmic pulsings from baby hiccups. In those moments, feel the sensations and know you are feeling them.

5. Take time every day to notice the natural world. While structured activities that put us in direct relationship to nature can be nourishing, like gardening, walking in the park, or going for a hike, the natural world is available to us any time we choose to take notice. This needn't be something we save for the weekend or when we "have time." Whenever we venture outside a building we have an opportunity to be in relationship to the natural world. Even on a rainy or snowy day, when we spend most of our time indoors, we can still use our eyes to be in relationship to nature as we look out the window. The same is true in an urban environment: you can always take a moment to look at the sky. Notice its color, and the clouds or lack of them. Let the infinite vastness of the sky above help put things into perspective, expanding your awareness beyond whatever particular human drama may be temporarily preoccupying your mind.

You may find that if you spend time in nature when you are pregnant, becoming more aware of Horticultural Time— the natural rhythms of the earth, its cycles of beginnings and endings, of the seasons, and of the changing balance between night and day— you may come to feel more connected to your growing baby and the life-giving process taking place within your body, gaining insight into how you are embedded in the larger whole of nature itself.

6. When you do any form of physical activity that you usually think of as exercise— walking, jogging, swimming, or working out at the gym— do it mindfully. One of the most memorable articles I read in nursing school many years ago was "The Hazards of Bed Rest," which documented how being in bed for any length of time negatively affects every organ of the body. Lungs can't fully inflate because of the pressure of the bed against the back; kidneys can't filter as well as they do when the body is upright; muscles begin to atrophy from lack of use. The take-home lesson for me was that our entire body functions optimally when we are active. Our bodies evolved to move.

While we have succeeded in making our lives easier and more convenient in many ways, that ease has come with a decrease in the number of minutes we actually move our bodies each day, which takes a toll on our general health. To make up for our more sedentary ways, we have to find time to exercise. But even while exercising we are often still not fully living in our bodies. Rather than being exactly where we are, feeling our feet moving on the treadmill or the muscles in our arms contracting and releasing as we move a machine or lift weights, we focus on a TV screen or on data from the exercise equipment or on reading a book or a magazine, thereby increasing the distance between the mind and body instead of promoting fully embodied presence. So whenever you are doing anything physical (which of course is all the time because you are alive), pay attention to the body. The payoff is huge.

7. Decrease stimulation of your eyes and ears, and increase your awareness of silence.

These days we often unthinkingly click on or crank up, subjecting our eyes and ears to a constant barrage of sights and sounds from our first waking moment until the moment we fall asleep. And when we do choose to listen to music, watch TV, get on the computer, or turn to our smartphones, what are we actually taking in, and at what volume? Are we really listening, or are we just turning on our electronic noisemakers out of habit or fear of being alone? Our nervous systems evolved in a much quieter world than the urban environment many of us live in today. If you haven't yet made silence a friend, you're missing something wonderful. If there is not enough silence in your life, add some in. Mindfulness practice can put us in touch with the simple yet profound pleasures of silence. It is here that we may find peace.

There is great power in the way that we think. Studies have proven that people with an optimistic and generally positive attitude are more successful in life and their careers. Negative thought patterns affect a person's ability to succeed and their mental health. Below is a list of traits of negative thinking. While reading these consider that as a person thinks this way they are internalizing these thought patterns. Remember you become what you dwell on.

How Negative People Think

Complain about what their life looks like but do not know how they want to change it.

They blame other people and circumstances for what has gone wrong instead of taking responsibility for themselves.

They feel powerless and that they have no control over their lives.

They believe the worst will always happen.

They use the words 'try' and 'I can't' instead of the words 'I can' and 'I will'

They always have an excuse why they 'can't' do something

They wander through life aimlessly, just waiting for life to happen to them

How Positive People Think

They know what they want and will work to obtain their goals.

They remain in control over their lives. They do not allow others to control them

When things don't go according to their plan, they do not give up or feel discouraged. Instead, they pick themselves back up and know that they can succeed still.

They have a balanced view of life and believe the best. They listen to positive input.

They do not use the words 'I can't' instead they will say 'I choose to do' or 'I choose not to do'. They always take control of their choices.

They are committed to staying positive

Have a list of goals that they are committed to working to attain.

They understand that in order to get the things they want out of life, they have to be committed to their goals and work hard. They do not resent the hard work instead it motivates them.

They know what they get out of life is a direct result of what they put into life

Ways to Think Positively

Look for opportunities

Stay focused on your positive goals and remove anything negative from your life that gets in the way of those goals

Look for the positive things in life and focus on them.

Positive thinking attracts positive results.

Stay flexible. Keep your options open.

Look for opportunities

Do not allow other's negativity to bring you down

Be open to new ideas

Act quickly

Keep a good sense of humor

- Stay objective. Rationally evaluate the facts of a situation rather than have your judgment clouded by emotions

- Believe in yourself

- Trust your instincts

- Take control and take responsibility

- Evaluate what is going on in a situation

- Consider the positives of every situation

- Focus on what you are thankful for

- Find the humor in every situation

- Find a role model and consider how they would react in your situation

- Consider what you have control over

- Release that which you cannot control

- Focus on what you need right now

- Think about how your actions are interpreted by others

- Consider carefully who and what you put your time and attention into

- Believe in yourself and your abilities

- Trust your instincts

Chapter 7

Relaxation

Often at the end of pregnancy, women are eager to meet their baby. They are reaching the end of this chapter with their body in full bloom. It is at this point that they may feel like their body is no longer theirs and they are eager for baby to make an appearance. If the due date is looming, or perhaps it has passed, their patience might be running out and so they look for ways to induce labour naturally.

A hypnobirthing course will teach you a number of tips and tricks to help you do that. None of these are harmful to you or your baby, so giving them a go is totally fine, but remember sometimes babies don't pay any attention to your impatience and they will keep you waiting a little bit longer…

For labour to begin, the conditions need to be ripe. Just think of our friends in the animal kingdom. They give birth when:

Nature decides that their baby is ready

They are in a safe space

When they know they will be uninterrupted

We humans need to have this reassurance too. So a mum needs to feel ready — not only emotionally, but in every other sense too — and she will probably want to be close to home as the estimated due date approaches, reassured that what she needs for labour and birth is close by.

What starts labour off is still a bit of a mystery. There are various theories out there, but what the definitive trigger is, is still unclear.

However, when all is well, a spontaneous labour tends to come on gradually.

The contractions are short in duration, spaced far apart and not too regular. As time passes and labour progresses, the contractions last longer, become more frequent and regular, and the intensity is likely to build.

For some women, spontaneous labour starts before their babies have reached full term and of course worries will immediately surface as to why this has happened and what will unfold. The best course of action in this situation is to get to hospital and let the professionals keep an eye on you and your baby.

Worrying too much and holding on to tension will not allow your body to work efficiently and help your baby descend. There are a number of ways to help you stay relaxed and comfortable, which enable your body to work powerfully and help birth your baby with more ease, such as breathing techniques and visualisations.

A hypnobirthing course will teach you these natural ways to stay relaxed, focused and comfortable in labour, to ensure that you are working with your body and your baby in the optimal way, and to help you have the best possible birth experience for the two of you.

Chapter 8

Preparing Your Baby And Body For Birth

Today, there are so many offers on the market that many expectant mothers feel overwhelmed and do not know what to do.

There is basically no right or wrong. Each method has its right to help a woman more or less. However, I have found nothing that has really helped every woman. The most important decision in birth preparation is: with whom I surround myself and how I influence these people, be it positive or negative!

As enriching and positive the exchange of pregnant women can/could be, the more vulnerable and negative it can be on the other side. You definitely ask yourself what should be negative for a pregnant group?

The explanation is quite simple: Here women come from different life situations, first-time and already experienced mothers. Each of these women bring their own story and in most cases, this leads to more uncertainty than self-assurance and support. All their own bad stories and those of the family, friends and acquaintances are told.

Every birth is different and something very personal. It is felt differently by every woman and many mothers tend to exaggerate, unfortunately, in your birth reports. It is important that you listen to yourself and learn to listen to your inner voice. During pregnancy, during birth and even later. In many books and articles on natural birth, the influence of positive thinking on the pain and the course of birth has already been reported.

This is nothing new, but a point that plays an important role in today's network with all the information overload.

You and your baby, are the main people and you should be able to go into childbirth untroubled and joyful. Less information is more in this case. There is no reason to be afraid or let yourself be unsettled. Nature has arranged it so that you can have an easy birth. The best way to do this is to keep you from all the negative stories.

Do not listen to all the other women, the media and what all the people in your environment want to tell you. Just add your favorite. This also applies to doctors: they are not omniscient and any theory, study and investigation can also be wrong.

I want to show you how you can differentiate, what your inner voice tells you and what feelings come from your subconscious mind.

As a future mother, you will have to trust your gut feeling more than ever before in your life. Your baby cannot tell you what's going on when it cries. It helps you tremendously when you learn to trust your feelings. Otherwise, you will study books and articles for hours on end and will not know what to do.

This insecurity can drive you crazy! You will run from one guidebook to the other and never feel right. But your baby needs your strength and self-assurance. If you are weak and helpless - how does your child feel?

You are the mama who is to give shelter. This starts with the pregnancy. Every woman is born by nature to be a good mother. You do not have to learn because you have everything in you. That is wonderful!

Just learn to pause and listen. Without external influences. You will master it, like millions of other women before you. The best preparation for the birth is, therefore, to listen to your inner voice. Another point that is at least as important is the contact with your child. This bond is so incredibly important for a smooth birth. You also give your baby the security to follow its natural instinct.

For optimal birth preparation, of course, you also have to think about where you want to release and who is to accompany you. You should make this decision all by yourself for yourself. You are the main person and you need more than ever security, as well as sureness. I know how difficult it can be in this decision not to be influenced by the outside. Every family member, friends, doctors and acquaintances want to give well-meaning advice. Girlfriends want to convince you of their clinic, homebirth or midwife. I recommend you make a basic decision here, whether you want to go to the hospital or not. The difference between a birth center and a homebirth is not particularly large. Make yourself neutral, without any of the stories you have ever heard with the following questions:

Can I feel comfortable in the hospital? When I think of my birth, do I feel more comfortable in the familiar/ domestic environment?

Do I trust doctors or midwives and alternative methods of healing?

Is it important for me to be in the hospital after the birth?

Can I relax in the clinic?

Do I want to go through birth alone with a midwife familiar to me?

Of course, you can trust that nothing happens and everything goes well. But you have to be 100% sure. If you have the confidence and the feeling it is right, then everything will be fine. I know that just at more than 3 births the probability of the uterus not closing completely and the risk of losing more blood is increasing. I do not feel that this will be the case. My inner voice feels more comfortable to have the safety of medical care nearby.

The birth is still very medical here and the clinics often have a standard as in Germany 30 years ago. The rate of PDA's is extremely high and you have women being strapped to the bed only 10 years ago!

Birth areas sometimes look like an operating room. There is no rooming-in, alternative birth positions and its aids. That did not make my search for the right hospital easy! Thankfully, a private clinic has opened a completely new "alternative birthplace" two months before my due date.

They even make a waterbirth possible, which is not to be found on the island. I love water and for me it is a big must. Another important point for me was to find the possibility that only one midwife, whom I trust, will look after me during the whole birth.

A good midwife can give you so much strength and become a true companion through birth. This costs a lot of strength and nerves.

This relaxation is immensely important. So, take all the time in the world and do not make quick decisions. Find the place where you feel comfortable and the people from whom you can trust one hundred percent.

There are only a few situations where you have no decision and you have to birth in a hospital. However, this is very rare. If you have a tendency, get information from both directions. Unfortunately, horror stories and anxiety are often widespread when it comes to the subject of homebirth.

Do not let yourself be deceived. I could also tell you some bad stories of mistakes of doctors and midwives in hospitals. The risk of something unexpected happening in the homebirth is very low. For this, we have the modern technology and homebirth midwifes with a lot of experience, which in the case of a danger of the homebirth do not agree or break off.

The person who accompanies you during the birth is another point that I would like to briefly describe. If you do not have a life partner who comes along, look for a person who knows you well and are with you on the same wavelength. Someone with whom you are medically and emotionally similar too. This does not always mean finding someone in your family. You should trust this person and this person also should be able to give you strength. The worst are people in a birth that need more attention and care than you do.

You cannot change your partner, but you know him and his behavior and views. Discuss everything in detail. It is important that you clearly define your wishes and also clearly communicate them to him. Make a plan of birth and thoughts on how you want his support.

A birth is never planable, but it is helpful if your environment knows what is important to you. If you do not want to give birth at home, think about what a home feeling can convey. Perhaps you want certain candles, scented oils, music or your favourite pillow? Think about things that will relax you and give you a feeling of well-being.

Relaxation is one of the most important things in pregnancy and that's why I created a special gift for you.

Chapter 9

Choosing Where To Give Birth

At some point fairly early on in your pregnancy your midwife should talk to you about your options about where you would like to give birth to your baby. If this has not happened, you can request to go through it at your next appointment.

You can give birth at home, or in a midwife-led unit (otherwise known as a 'birth centre', or 'home from home') or in the main delivery unit (labour ward). Midwife-led units may be either freestanding (not attached to a hospital – though this is unlikely in the UK) or alongside (in the same building as the main labour ward – more usual).

It is well worth doing some research around each of the options discussed below. After all, when you plan a holiday chances are you spend at least a little (probably a lot!) of time researching your accommodation, or the resort.

Or, if you were planning a wedding, you would likely spend a fair amount of time planning and looking into the venue and making sure it suited your needs.

So take the time to research one of the biggest things you will ever do – have a baby.

You can compare different maternity statistics unit by unit by visiting http://www.which.co.uk/birth-choice

If you don't know your options you don't have any.

Home birth

Some women like the idea of giving birth at home – a place where they are in control and feel less like a patient, are able to have a bath, and to eat and drink whatever and whenever they want. It is easier to distract yourself at home and carry on as normal for longer. You can book a home birth with your midwife. When you go into labour you call your midwife and she or a member of her team, who you likely will already know or have met, will come out to you at home. When the birth is imminent, she will usually call a second midwife to help her. If you book a home birth you can change your mind at any time during your pregnancy, even during labour and instead opt to go to the birth centre or labour ward.

What are the benefits of a home birth?

If you plan a home birth you are more likely to in advance have met the midwife who will take care of you during your labour (if your homebirth team offer what is called 'case loading' - where a named midwife will provide continuity of care). This can help you feel more comfortable and relaxed. Research has shown that labour usually progresses well at home when a woman knows her midwife.

You are in your own domain, free to move as you wish and eat and drink whatever you fancy, whenever you fancy.

If you need to transfer into hospital, your midwife will go with you. She may stay, or she may hand you over to the care of the hospital midwives on duty.

There is less pressure to labour within a particular time-frame, which means that fewer interventions are offered to speed up your labour.

Should you require medical intervention your midwife will arrange for you to go to your local hospital.

There is less risk of infection at a home birth.

You really do get one-to-one care, as the midwife will be focusing on you and your baby, no one else. She will be regularly listening in to your baby's heartbeat and will not hesitate to suggest you transfer in if she suspects there is a problem – something she will do long before any situation becomes an emergency.

Home birth is strongly associated with improved breastfeeding outcomes.

Midwives are highly skilled and trained to deal with emergencies.

Home birth and safety

Medical emergencies can occur anywhere, regardless of where a woman gives birth – but do remember that giving birth is generally very safe.

Midwives are highly skilled and trained to deal with any urgent situations whilst calling for further help. For example, if a post-partum haemorrhage were to happen, the midwife would have the initial drugs necessary to manage this and would arrange prompt transfer into hospital.

In some cases women requesting a home birth may be encouraged to give birth in hospital, for example in the event of a pregnancy lasting longer than 42 weeks, or the baby being in a breech position. Some women with less straightforward pregnancies or less usual factors to consider choose to research the pros and cons of their specific situation and make an informed decision to still give birth at home.

What's available at a home birth?

You can have a water birth at home if you hire a pool. Sometimes you can find second-hand ones online, and just buy a new liner. Your home birth team may have a pool you can hire.

You can hire or buy a TENS machine and use this.

You will have access to gas and air.

You may have access to either pethidine or diamorphine (opiods).

NICE guidance states that you should be supported and informed about your birth place options. Your GP or midwife should not try to dissuade you from your choice unless they feel there is a genuine medical reason. If there is medical reason as to why something is being suggested then of course you'd be wise to discuss this and ask for sources of research and information

69

on it. But the decision is always yours and you are free to make your own choices even if your caregivers do not agree with you.

Birth centre

Sometimes a birth centre is referred to as 'home from home' or 'midwife led suite'. Giving birth in a birth centre can be a great option for many women who have had straightforward pregnancies. Birth centres are run by midwives and do not routinely use medical interventions if labour progresses well. As many labours progress well, birth centres are a good alternative to giving birth in hospital.

Should a woman require any medical intervention she can transfer to the labour ward. Most birth centres are in the same building, even the same floor, as the main hospital/labour ward, which many women find reassuring.

Pros of using a birth centre

Birth centres feel more homely and less clinical, which in turn can make you feel more relaxed.

They are often more spacious, with more equipment available, such as birthing stools, birth balls and padded floors to comfortably kneel on.

They may have a double bed available for after the birth for your birth partner to stay overnight, but this is sometimes tucked out of the way or folded up against the wall to encourage women not to hop up on it! This is because research shows that being upright and mobile during active labour has many benefits, shortening labour and making it feel more manageable.

Within birth centres birth is seen as a normal event rather than a risky one, and having a straightforward birth is much more likely. Straightforward birth means giving birth vaginally, without any procedures or interventions such as assisted birth (forceps or ventouse), induction of labour or caesarean birth.

Some centres allow you to stay in the room, with your partner and baby, for your whole stay, though you will need to transfer out if someone wants to use the room. Others request that you transfer to the postnatal ward at some point after the birth.

The midwives who work in a birth centre have often chosen this environment as they have a passionate interest in supporting women to birth with little or no intervention.

Cons of using a birth centre

If you decide you want an epidural you need to transfer to the labour ward. If your birth centre is not located within the hospital, ask your midwife which unit you would transfer to and how long this would take.

What's available at a birth centre?

Very often pools are plumbed in or inflatable ones are available.

You can hire or buy a TENS machine and use this.

You will have access to entonox (gas and **air).**

Sometimes the midwives are trained in and can offer aromatherapy massage or reflexology.

Often you will be able to have pethidine or diamorphine for pain relief during labour should you want this.

There is less equipment visible, which helps to give a feel of birth being a normal event.

If your baby needed special care they would be transferred to the special care baby unit, which in most cases will be in the same building.

While the transfer may not happen instantly unless it is an emergency, you can always change your mind and transfer out of the birth centre and onto the labour ward should you wish to – for example if you decided you now wanted an epidural (epidurals are not available on the birth centre).

Hospital birth/labour ward

Some women choose to give birth on the labour ward as they find it reassuring.

If a woman is having consultant led care she may be more likely to be offered the labour ward rather than the birth centre.

However, being in the hospital environment makes it more likely that you will be offered interventions, which is something to bear in mind. There is also less privacy in a hospital setting.

If you have had a complicated pregnancy or are likely to require a caesarean birth for medical reasons, you will be encouraged to give birth in hospital, on the labour ward.

Your care will still be provided by midwives, but doctors will be available if required. It is unlikely that you will have met your midwife in advance of your birth.

What is available on the labour ward?

You will have access to an epidural, pethidine/diamorphine and entonox (gas and air).

Some labour wards have birthing pools available – ask your midwife or check the Which? Birth website to see if bringing your own pool in is an option.

Access to a special care baby unit.

Some women like to start in the birth centre and transfer to the labour ward if they feel they would like an epidural. Once you are in your room on the labour ward you can make it your own. You may like to:

Dim the lights as low as you can.

Cover windows with blackout blinds.

Bring battery-operated fairy lights for a beautiful, soft glow.

Cover any unused equipment with a scarf or blanket/towel to make it feel less clinical.

Birth balls should be provided but you can bring your own.

Raise or lower the bed so you are not tempted to get on it and not move around much thereafter.

Bring music.

Bring an essential oil of your choice to breathe in from a piece of fabric.

Cover the clock so you are not focused on it.

Chapter 10

Packing The Birth Bag

Some people like to pack two bags, one for labour and one for after the birth. It is a good idea for your birth partner to have their own bag too with a change of clothes, toiletries and snacks in (so they're not taking your stash!). If you are driving to the hospital or birth centre you could then leave the postnatal bag in the boot of the car, to save room.

A good tip is to lay out everything for your labour and birth bag on the bed and ask your partner to pack it. That way he or she will know exactly where everything is.

You will probably only use a few things that you bring, but as it can be hard to know what those things will be, packing for most eventualities is normal! Pack enough for one night. If you need more, your partner or a friend can go home and get things for you.

Here are some suggestions to consider:

Your maternity notes if they are still the hand-held version.

Several copies of your birth preferences sheet – you can stick one up on the wall too (bring sticky tack if you want to do this).

A TENS machine with spare batteries and spare pads.

Food – a selection of sweet and savoury items for you and your birth partner. You never know what you might fancy. If you like bananas, these provide good energy, as would dried fruits. Food for after the birth is good too, just in case it's the middle of the night and nothing is open.

Sports cap water bottles or bendy straws so you can easily stay hydrated whatever position you are in.

Phone charger – if you use your phone as your camera this is especially important for those first pictures! Likewise if you use your mobile phone to listen to hypnobirthing downloads.

Phone numbers written down, in case the phone runs out and you are unable to charge it.

Camera if you're not planning on using your phone.

Toiletries.

Ear plugs.

A plain carrier oil or pregnancy massage oil for massages or putting a few drops of whatever smell you like (providing it is safe to inhale or have on your skin during labour) onto some fabric to aid relaxation. This is useful as if you get fed up with the aroma you can just remove the fabric.

Music to listen to, or if hypnobirthing, the relaxation MP3s if they are not already downloaded onto your mobile phone. If relevant, take a battery-operated machine (laptop or a way to play your MP3s or music playlist), in case you are unable to plug things in.

Things to make the environment as dark as possible – eye mask? Blackout blinds? The room is yours to change as you wish!

Water spray to keep cool.

A fan.

A loose, comfortable change of clothes for you.

Buy some cheap flannels, soak them in water and freeze them separately in sandwich bags. You can then take them out and use them on the back of your neck to cool you down.

A hot water bottle – some women find warmth comforting.

Dressing gown.

Slippers.

Socks.

Flip-flops for the shower (non-slip!).

A nightdress or big t-shirt.

Lip balm.

Hair band. If you have long hair, you might want it tied up.

Pillows in your own pillow cases – the familiar scent of home will be very comforting and far more comfortable than the starchy hospital ones. Use non-white cases so the staff know the pillows are yours from home.

Wipes for a quick freshen-up.

Toiletries for a longer freshen-up! Treat yourself to a luxurious soap or shower gel. Just brushing your teeth can help to refresh you.

A towel.

Postnatal bag

Loose comfortable clothing for going home in.

Nursing bra and breast pads.

Maternity pads – you will likely need around 3-4 packets of these as they will require changing around every 2-3 hours for the first couple of days or so. Postnatal bleeding is normal and healthy after birth, whether caesarean or vaginal.

Old or cheap, large and comfortable underwear.

Hair brush.

Pyjamas/something to relax in.

Clothes for your baby such as a hat, a couple of all in one stretchy outfits, a cardigan, a couple of vests.

A night shirt that opens at the front for easy skin to skin contact with your baby when feeding him.

Baby blanket and/or snowsuit if the weather is cold.*

Socks and or booties (depending on the weather).

Nappies.

Car seat in the car, already practised with or installed and ready to go!

***Remember to always remove bulky clothing before putting your baby into his or her car seat. If it is cold, you can tuck a blanket over the car seat straps once they are secured correctly.

***It is well worth getting your car seat checked to ensure that it is fitted correctly, as many are not and are therefore useless. There are independent car seat specialists, or sometimes local councils offer a free car sear checking service.

Chapter 11

Basic Hypnobirthing Techniques

RELAXATION (AND RELAXATION TECHNIQUES)

Join a huge number of moms overall who have found the delights of a quiet loosened up birth.

Why learn at a class?

You'll get the chance to meet other hopeful guardians and offer encounters with them.

You will work with a certified expert and as a trance inducer and hypnobirthing educator I will show you the strategies of spellbinding such that works for you I can tell the best way to utilize the procedures as viably as conceivable during pregnancy and past and you will have the chance to pose the same number of inquiries as you like and have the option to rehearse your new aptitudes.

There is center around both you and your accomplice with the goal that you are similarly engaged with the birth procedure. This incorporates post natal help too with an emphasis on you as guardians yet in addition on the uncommon family associations that are major in sound connections.

To what extent is the regimen?

The regimen is part into 4 week by week sessions and expenses £295 per couple.

The following regimen begins on ninth September 2019 and there will be extra regimens running consistently. I additionally offer 121 sessions and private ends of the week for Hypnobirthing just as private hypnotherapy for any part of your life

Progressive relaxation

Unwinding systems for torment the executives in labor

What is the issue?

This Cochrane Review saw whether mind-body systems for unwinding, for example, breathing procedures, representation, yoga or music would help with decreasing agony, and improve ladies' encounters of work. We gathered and examined every important examination to respond to this inquiry.

For what reason is this significant?

The agony of work can be serious, with body pressure, nervousness and dread exacerbating it. Numerous ladies might want to experience work without utilizing drugs, or obtrusive strategies, for example, an epidural. These ladies frequently go to correlative treatments to decrease the power of agony in labor and improve their encounters of work.

Numerous corresponding treatments are utilized by ladies in labor, including needle therapy, mind-body strategies, knead, reflexology, natural drugs or homeopathy, spellbinding, music and fragrant healing. Mind-body systems for unwinding can be broadly available to ladies through the instructing of these procedures during antenatal classes. The unwinding strategies incorporate guided symbolism, dynamic unwinding and breathing systems. We additionally remember yoga and music for this audit. Other Cochrane Reviews spread trance in labor, manual techniques (like back rub and reflexology), fragrance based treatment and needle therapy/pressure point massage. Huge numbers of these unwinding systems are adapting techniques used to diminish the experience of agony. These strategies use rehearses that plan to decrease pressure and lessen the view of agony. It is critical to inspect if these treatments work and are sheltered, to empower ladies to settle on educated choices about their consideration.

What proof did we find?

We discovered 15 investigations including 1731 ladies that contributed information to the examinations. Studies were embraced over the world, remembering nations for Europe and Scandinavia, and Iran, Taiwan, Thailand, Turkey and USA.

We found that unwinding strategies, yoga and music may assist ladies with overseeing work torment, in spite of the fact that the nature of the proof differed among low and low, and more information are required. Likewise, in these preliminaries there were varieties in how these methods were utilized. There was no unmistakable proof that these treatments affected helped vaginal or cesarean birth. There were deficient information to state if these strategies affected the child's condition during childbirth.

The utilization of some unwinding treatments, yoga, or music may potentially be useful with lessening the force of agony, and in helping ladies feel more in charge and happy with their works. In any case, the wide varieties in kinds of strategies utilized in these examinations make it hard to state explicitly what may support ladies. In this manner further research contemplates are required.

Disappearing letters

HypnoBirthing- The Mongan Method - is a finished antenatal program that shows straightforward however explicit self-spellbinding, unwinding and breathing strategies for pregnancy and birth.

Felicity Lamb, 27, is mum to Bernie, nine months. She working on HypnoBirthing methods all through her pregnancy and effectively utilized them to deal with her torment in labor.

How could you get some answers concerning HypnoBirthing?

My generally excellent companion Zoe chose to do a HypnoBirthing regimen after she attempted it when she was pregnant with her first infant. She disclosed to me how loosening up it could be. At that point, when my companion Jen took it up, I thought - I must discover more. So Jen loaned me a book and CD, and I took it from that point.

What strategies did you realize?

I took in a great deal. The Rainbow Relaxation Technique - where you picture objects of various hues thusly, for example, water for blue and a cornfield for yellow - was extremely useful and should be possible with the CD. The music is magnificent and truly carries your musings into agreement with the characteristic progression of vitality inside your own body.

The 'certifications for simpler, open to birthing' truly helped me through the birth experience itself. Insistences are sure words or expressions that are rehashed to help trigger the intuitive personality without hesitation, anything from "I believe my body and I pursue its lead" to "My infant moves delicately along its adventure". I read my picked expressions day by day all through pregnancy, I felt it was best when I said them for all to hear in my room - it truly helped me to acknowledge I could do it.

Light touch massage

Discharge Your Natural Painkillers Through the Light Touch Massage

From time to time, when we need to unwind in the wake of a monotonous seven day stretch of work, we get a back rub. Attempt to recall the last time you had a back rub. How could you feel? Did you feel somewhat woozy? Did you likewise feel without a care in the world?

We as a whole might want to get a back rub now and again, in light of the fact that a back rub discharges endorphins into our circulation system. These endorphins are regular hormones that are more strong than morphine with regards to diminishing sensations and our view of agony.

That implies that inside our body is a characteristic painkiller that is activated by contact. Our body discharges endorphins because of solid sensations as a way to control them. Our endorphins travel through our nerves right from the mind.

Endorphins and Pain

The arrival of endorphins by the nerves restrains a few or the entirety of the torment messages going up to the cerebrum. For some ladies, endorphins will likewise emphatically change the memory of their introduction to the world experience and sometimes actuate an amnesic, fantastic impact.

Without the dangerous reactions of epidurals and medicinal mediation during birthing, endorphins is one of the key factors in having a dauntless and effortless birth that is quiet, simple, and snappy.

Attempt to review snapshots of affection making with your accomplice. Didn't light contacts send a rush to your body, making you feel somewhat unsteady or even sleepy? That is the intensity of contacts influencing our nerves, and sending endorphins to our whole body.

A back rub, in the mean time, diminishes the pulse, brings down circulatory strain, and expands blood regimen and lymph stream, loosens up muscles, improves scope of feelings, and, in particular for birthing, builds endorphins.

Ladies in birth are, now and again, unreasonably touchy for profound back rubs, so a light touch knead is the most ideal approach to actuate these agony desensitizing hormones.

Light Touch Massage Technique:

While the Light Touch Massage is the most ideal approach to discharge endorphins to help make birthing simpler and more quiet, few out of every odd mum-to-be will like this method. Some will lean toward an alternate sort of back rub, so you should rehearse this was an accomplice, and attempt to check your response to the back rub.

The Light Touch Massage is only one of the numerous apparatuses in the Hypnobirthing Hub Regimens you can use to make your introduction to the world simpler, more quiet, and effortless. For more practice on the Light Touch Massage, you can watch the video exhibition.

Anchors

A stay is a physical relationship with an inclination. These obviously can be negative or positive however we focus on the positive in hypnobirthing. The tune was a grapple for me and raised how I was feeling at the time. Stays are an incredible asset to use in hypnobirthing. They can be something you see, hear, smell, taste, feel or contact.

By working on hypnobirthing you can make grapples which will bring sentiments of quiet, unwinding, wellbeing, certainty and trust during birth. These can be shaped from numerous points of view. Insistences, contact and back rub, hypnobirthing unwinding MP3S, fragrant healing oils, home solaces, for example, a most loved pad or cover and pictures are altogether utilized in readiness to plant stays in your psyche, which will achieve positive emotions you can reproduce and draw after during birth.

These not just make a real physical reaction in your body, for example, keeping your muscles loose, your breathing profound and moderate, your pulse and circulatory strain unfaltering yet additionally a ground-breaking passionate reaction in your brain as well. So that anyway you birth your child you will connect it with sentiments of energy, serenity and bliss.

Working on breathing methods during pregnancy is a major grapple for unwinding. Simply going through five minutes daily will have a significant effect. Include a most loved smell and music to the blend and you will have yourself three ground-breaking stays, that will assist you with feeling loose and quiet on the enormous day. These can be utilized after birth as well! Whatever positive affiliation you have made with them will return flooding, making you feel loose, focused and more grounded.

 Here is a short unwinding activity for you, that your can rehearse whenever and anyplace! Appreciate it!

Ensure you are sitting serenely and safely.

Start breathing profoundly in through the nose and a more drawn out breath out through the mouth. Close your eyes.

Envision the air going up through the nose and down into your lungs. Spot your hands on your mid-region, feel the air growing your ribs and arriving at your child.

On the out breath you can feel your jaw, tongue and shoulders unwind. Increasingly more with every breath. You can see your infant nestled into and cheerful inside you.

Rehash a couple of times in your brain - I feel loose, I let go of strain and I confide during the time spent birth.

Open your eyes and rehash a couple of breaths to change in accordance with the present time and place.

Breathing Techniques

Diminishing sensations during labor can make your introduction to the world simpler, faster, and more settled, yet is this really conceivable? It is! You can decrease sensations during your works with the correct breathing systems.

With the information and apparatuses that will assist you with taking advantage of your characteristic abilities and mental activities, you can experience your floods smoothly and effectively. Fortunately, the Hypnobirthing Hub breathing procedures can help you through your floods or withdrawals, giving you more solace, quiet, and power during your work.

To what extent would you be able to inhale submerged? Thirty seconds? An entire minute? For a significant number of us, holding our breath submerged is a troublesome task. Numerous competitors and great swimmers or jumpers, however, can hold their breath for seven minutes or longer submerged.

How would they even do that? That is on the grounds that they increment their lung limit and inhale profoundly into their midriff. Don't you wish you could do that?

Luckily, with enough practice and tutelage, you can. Why? This is on the grounds that you'd have to inhale profoundly to loosen up your muscles and leave your uterus free of strain. This will assist you with taking care of and oversee agony and worry during your introduction to the world.

Through the Hypnobirthing Hub, you will become familiar with the correct breathing systems to deal with your floods and to reduce your agony during birth. This sort of breathing will likewise build cervix widening, which will decrease your birthing time.

Hypnobirthing Hub Breathing Technique Surge Breathing Infographic

Stomach Breathing

The point when you experience your floods or withdrawals, you don't need to remember muddled strategies. You just need to recall breathing examples that are now normal to your body.

Flood breathing is stomach relaxing. All through each flood, you have to inhale equally and profoundly, breathing down into your midriff, feeling it rise and grow.

In unwinding breathing, you figure out how to quiet yourself, and it doesn't make a difference where you inhale into. In flood breathing, it's critical to inhale into your stomach or guts. There are a few people who regularly inhale into their bellies. There are other people who inhale into their chests. Thus, it's critical to watch your breathing examples.

Do this speedy exercise: Place one hand on your chest, and another on your stomach. Unwind as much as you can, and put power or exertion into your relaxing. Simply see where your breathing goes.

On the off chance that you routinely profound into your chest, your rib confine agreements and it requires you more vitality and exertion to move those ribs upward. Along these lines, during a flood, when you inhale into your gut, your breath gets increasingly slow. You use less vitality and get more oxygen. The more oxygen you inhale into your tummy through the flood, the better for you, your muscles, and your infant.

Decrease of Stress

At the point when you do flood breathing, you extend your mid-region and lungs, which gives the vertical muscles of your uterus more space to reach down and pull up the roundabout muscles. This additional space for your uterus muscles decreases the power of the flood and makes it simpler to oversee.

The more you inhale into your belly, the simpler the weight impressions of the flood will be for you. Try not to be scared by stomach breathing in case you're accustomed to breathing into your chest. Have you seen resting babies of late? They inhale with their stomaches. Stomach breathing will come to you normally. You simply need some training.

Here's How (Surge Breathing Technique):

Spot your fingers simply addressing your paunch button (only the center fingers will contact).

Take a long, slow and full breath in through your nose into your mid-region, breathing up as far you can.

As you take in your fingers will fall apart (the more profound the breath, the more remote away your fingers will turn into).

At that point gradually inhale out through your mouth as your fingers come back to the simply contacting once more.

Gradually take in for whatever length of time that you can to arrive at an agreeable number, maybe 10? (Try not to hold your breath!! You and your infant need oxygen.)

Gradually inhale out to a similar check.

Gradually take in 1,2,3,4,5,6,7,8,9,10 (or what feels directly for you).

Gradually inhale out 1,2,3,4,5,6,7,8,9,10 (or what feels directly for you).

Keep on taking along these lines for five in and out breaths.

Adapt free hypnobirthing methods video exhibits or join our classes at Manly to rehearse flood relaxing. Planning can help go far to make your introduction to the world simpler. You can look at our hypnobirthing free assets and best hypnobirthing sound manual for start your voyage to a more settled and superb birth.

CALM BREATHING

Hypnobirthing Hub Breathing Techniques: Relaxation Breathing

It is anything but an unprecedented sight for an anticipating that mum should frenzy and feel terrified of work, particularly a first-time mum who has heard every one of the anecdotes about agonizing births. Normally, when she begins shouting, the specialist or medical caretaker says, "Relax. Simply relax. You have to quiet down."

At the point when you're pushed or apprehensive, it's never simple to quiet down, to unwind, and to inhale appropriately. It's troublesome, yet not feasible. With hypnobirthing, you can unwind and inhale tranquilly to remove the weight from your body, to lighten the torment during work.

With the Hypnobirthing Hub, you can utilize unwinding breathing methods, which will assist you with resisting the urge to panic and loose during your pregnancy, through your floods, and during your work. This sort of breathing procedure is perfect for the beginning times or pre-work stages and in the middle of floods to enable you to unwind. The more you unwind, the more your muscles will extricate, the simpler your work will be.

Unwinding breathing is something beyond working on breathing in and breathing out. All in all, how is it done? Do this short exercise:

Close your eyes, a take a long breath in and afterward a long breath out. Do you discover the in-breath or out-breath all the more unwinding?

Since out-breathing or breathing out is all the more unwinding, you will concentrate on this more when you do unwinding relaxing. Your out-breath will be twice the length of your in-breath.

Unwinding Between Your Surges

In the middle of your compressions is when dread and uneasiness sneaks in. Indeed, even a spur of the moment remark questioning your capacity to deal with the floods, or a doubting glance toward you can make you begin to feel terrified and on edge.

Since we birth like well evolved creatures and have such a basic reaction at our birthing time, our impulses are excessively elevated and we feel extremely delicate as of now.

You can't control everybody and everything around you during your introduction to the world, yet you can control your very own feelings and make a feeling of quiet at whatever point you need it. In the event that you ever feel you could do with some additional unwinding between your floods, simply take a couple of unwinding breaths and feel restored and sure again.

Unwinding Breathing Technique

Enable your eyelids to delicately close.

Deliberately drop and loosen up your jaw, neck and entire body.

Gradually breathe in through your nose (or mouth) to the check of four (4). Take in 1,2,3,4

Gradually breathe out through your nose (or mouth) to the check of eight (8). Inhale out 1,2,3,4,5,6,7,8

Rehash multiple times or as expected to feel superbly loose.

It is likewise critical to recollect that this breathing is a delicate breathing procedure that spotlights on breathing basically from your upper chest (or whatever feels directly for you). It isn't explicitly stomach breathing, as in flood breathing, which you can find out about in our blog.

Keep in mind that careful discipline brings about promising results (or practically flawless). On the off chance that you need to feel increasingly loose and responsible for your introduction to the world, you can look into our Hypnobirthing Classes at Manly or download our Hypnobirthing Home Study Regimen Manual Downloads where you can tune in to our digital recordings and concentrate diverse breathing systems from our manual.

For an increasingly point by point and bit by bit direct on unwinding breathing strategies, look at our Hypnobirthing Relaxation Music, and consistently stay tuned to our blog!

Breathing Techniques, Hypnobirthing, Hypnosis

SURGE BREATHING

Designed Breathing During Labor: Techniques and Benefits

Designed breathing alludes to the demonstration of breathing at any number of potential rates and profundities. A few ladies incline toward breathing profoundly, utilizing their stomach to fill their guts with air. Other ladies incline toward light breathing, breathing in only enough to fill their chest. The objective is to discover breathing designs that have a quieting and loosening up impact. Your breathing ought to be at an agreeable rate and ought not make you feel shy of breath or unsteady.

The more you find out about work and birth, the more you will perceive how various examples of breathing are utilized at various stages. You will find out about utilizing breathing to concentrate on making every compression a beneficial piece of the birthing procedure. Regardless of whether pregnant or not, designed breathing is useful in adapting to different kinds of agony, inconvenience, tension, and dread.

Advantages of rehearsing designed relaxing

Breathing turns into a programmed reaction to torment

The mother stays in an increasingly loosened up state and will react all the more decidedly to the beginning of torment

The enduring musicality of breathing is quieting during work

Gives a feeling of prosperity and control

Expanded oxygen gives more quality and vitality to both the mother and child

Carries reason to every withdrawal, making constrictions progressively gainful

Designed breathing and unwinding can become strategies for managing life's consistently stressors

Step by step instructions to rehearse designed relaxing

Congested driving conditions, cerebral pains, and family unit tasks give chances to rehearse distinctive breathing methods and make them part of your everyday practice. To recreate work, some labor instructors recommend grasping an ice block while rehearsing compelling breathing methods.

Step by step instructions to start

Toward the start and end of every compression make sure to take a profound, purifying, loosening up breath. This hones your concentration as well as gives more oxygen to your infant, your muscles and your uterus.

Breathing designs for the principal phase of work:

Slow Breathing

Start moderate breathing when withdrawals are serious enough that you can never again walk or talk through them without stopping. Utilize moderate relaxing for whatever length of time that you think that its accommodating. Change to another example on the off chance that you become tense and can never again unwind during compressions.

Take a sorting out breath, a major murmur when the withdrawal starts. Discharge all pressure (go limp all finished – from head to toe) as you inhale out.

Concentrate.

Gradually breathe in through your nose and breathe out through your mouth, enabling all your air to stream out with a murmur. Respite until the air appears to "need" to come in once more.

With each breathe out, center around loosening up an alternate piece of your body (see Relaxation Techniques).

Light Accelerated Breathing

Take a sorting out breath—a major murmur when the compression starts. Discharge all pressure (go limp all finished – from head to toe) as you inhale out.

Concentrate.

Breathe in gradually through your nose and breathe out through your mouth. Quicken and help your breathing as the compression increments in force. On the off chance that the compression tops early, at that point you should quicken from the get-go in the constriction. It if tops all the more step by step, you will work up to top speed all the more gradually. Keep your mouth and shoulders loose.

As the withdrawal diminishes in force, continuously moderate your breathing rate, exchanging back to taking in through your nose and out through your mouth.

At the point when the compression closes, take your completing breath—breathe out with a murmur.

Variable (Transition) Breathing

This is a variety of light relaxing. It is in some cases alluded to as "gasp blow" or "hee-hee-who" relaxing. Variable breathing joins light shallow breathing with an occasional longer or increasingly articulated exhalation. Variable breathing is utilized in the principal organize in the event that you feel overpowered, incapable to unwind, despondently, or depleted.

Take a sorting out breath—a major murmur when the constriction starts. Discharge all pressure (go limp all finished – from head to toe) as you inhale out.

Concentrate on your accomplice or a point of convergence, for example, an image.

At the point when the withdrawal closes take a couple of profound loosening up breaths with a moan.

Breathing to abstain from pushing at an inappropriate time

There will be times all through the two phases of work when you will need to push or weigh down, however it isn't the ideal time. Most ladies need to hold their breath during these, especially troublesome minutes. Abstain from holding your breath by taking in and out continually or by raising your jaw and blowing or gasping. This shields you from adding to the pushing that your body is as of now doing.

Breathing designs for the second phase of work

Removal Breathing

Utilized once the cervix is completely enlarged and the second phase of work has started.

Take a sorting out breath—a major moan when the compression starts. Discharge all pressure (go limp all finished – from head to toe) as you inhale out.

Concentrate on the infant going disheartened, or on another positive picture.

Inhale gradually, giving the constriction a chance to control you. Quicken or help your breathing as vital for comfort. At the point when you can't fight the temptation to push (when it "requests" that you participate), take a major breath, fold your jaw to chest, twist your body and fit forward. At that point hunker down, while holding your breath or gradually discharging air by snorting or groaning. Generally significant of all, loosen up the pelvic floor. Help the child descend by discharging any pressure in the perineum.

Following 5-6 seconds, discharge your breath, at that point take in and out. At the point when the inclination to drive assumes control over participate by hunkering down. How hard you push is directed by your sensation. You will proceed along these lines until the constriction dies down. The desire to push travels every which way in waves during the compression. Utilize these breaks to inhale profoundly giving oxygen to your blood and child.

At the point when the compression closes, loosen up your body and take a couple of quieting breaths.

Birth breathing

All alone, the term trance signifies "a strategy during which an individual encounters proposed changes in sensation, observation, thought or conduct." One specific marked variant of mesmerizing during the birthing procedure is alluded to as HypnoBirthing.

While this fundamental thought has been around for quite a long time, the particular term was begat in the 1989 book HypnoBirthing: A Celebration of Life composed by trance inducer Marie Mongan. Her thoughts are affected by early "normal birth" defenders Dr. Jonathan Dye and Dr. Grantly Dick-Read.

At its center, HypnoBirthing expects to enable a lady to manage any dread or uneasiness she may have around birth. It includes different unwinding and self-mesmerizing procedures to help loosen up the body previously and during work and birth.

The thought is that when the body and brain are in a totally loosened up state, birth can happen all the more rapidly and effortlessly on the grounds that the body doesn't battle the characteristic procedure.

VISUALIZATION TECHNIQUE

3 Birth Visualizations To Rock Your Birth

You don't have to utilize them all. Various things claim to various individuals. Maybe simply pick a couple to rehearse?

At the point when the flood comes, envision a wave building. What's more, as the flood gets more grounded, the wave gets greater and greater and greater and greater until in the long run you arrive at the top and the wave falls away. Your on the opposite side. You did it. You're over that one. Furthermore, presently, you reset your psyche until the following one comes. Completely loose. Feeling appreciative that each wave is presenting to you a little closer to your little one. Your muscles work best when they are relaxed.Waves

Envision a goddess situated in front you. She is wonderful, focused and grounded. She is solid and incredible. Her ladylike vitality is divine. She is clear. She is YOU! Envision the vitality that runs however her goes through you too.goddess

At the point when the sensations get more grounded and you are beginning to need to inhale through them, the sensations you are believing are really your uterus is attracting up to enable your child to get out. In this way, one thought is on the in-breath you can envision in your mind bubbles rising and afterward as you inhale out gradually however your mouth, you may get a kick out of the chance to envision overwhelming the air pockets as they keep on skimming upwards .

101

Ultra-Deeping Techniques

Having an infant is one of life's most stunning endowments and having the option to make, sustain and birth new life is completely a wonder. However, when numerous ladies think about the idea of conceiving an offspring this frequently fills them with dread and frenzy. The media could be accused for this previously established inclination just as other people who share their terrible accounts of work and how agonizing the experience was. Does work truly need to be like this? Or then again is there another option?

Releasing Fear

Being able to release fears is a big part of hypnobirthing. When you listen to a negative birth story you add to or top up your 'birth mind library' with yet more negative stories. It may not seem like much at the time, but you can't 'un-hear' things that are said and your subconscious mind remembers it all. Now is the time to be solely focusing on preparing for a positive birth. Rather than watching or reading the news last thing at night, which is usually a less than relaxing experience, you could instead choose to listen to your hypnobirthing MP3 (most of the scripts later in this chapter are available to you as MP3s).

Watch a positive birth video, read some positive birth stories or join a hypnobirthing Facebook page such as **Baby Bumps – Hypnobirthing South London** to have your news feed full of supportive, positive birth stories and information.

Think about where your fears come from – are they actually your fears or just things that you have heard along the way? Birth is very safe for most women, but we tend to only remember the negative things we hear.

Write your concerns down, whether they are about birth or anything else that you want to release. Ask yourself "how likely is this to happen?", "is this my truth, or is it someone else's story?" If 'XYZ' is truly is on the cards for you, ask yourself "who can I talk to in order to gain some perspective on it all?" Sometimes the action of simply writing your fears down and/or talking it through with someone you trust, is enough to get it out of your head and make it feel a little less overwhelming.

If you still feel after honestly thinking about your fears, that they are very real for you, focus a lot of time on listening to the fear release script/MP3 (you can find this script later on in this chapter) and listen to this above the others until you start to feel a shift or change. You can also read other hypnobirthing books and saturate your brain with as many different sources of positive birth stories as is possible! If at all possible, attend a hypnobirthing course.

Consider seeing an experienced hypnotherapist if you feel that none of the above is helping you or you still feel stuck in fear.

Informed Decision Making

Labour and birth don't always go as expected and it's useful to keep a flexible outlook on it. Having said that, writing a birth preferences/birth plan is very important as it enables you to start thinking about your wishes for your birth and what you might want in other situations should your birth take a different turn. There is an example of a birth plan in this book.

Sometimes, during the course of a labour an unexpected complication may arise and your Midwife may suggest a way to proceed. Your midwife may ask how you feel about 'X, Y or Z' and it can be hard to know how best to go forward. It is, absolutely fine to let the Midwife know what your birth preferences are, and providing it is not an emergency situation (and it will be obvious if it is), you can ask as many questions as you want to. Asking questions can help you to gather information, feel involved and make informed decisions, rather than making decisions based around fear and the unknown, or feeling pushed into a decision without fully understanding it.

Different midwives have different approaches and, as wonderful as midwives are, they are only human and, like the rest of us, possibly have a preferred way of doing something – but there may be another way of achieving the same result, whatever it may be. It is always worthwhile asking questions. Below are some suggestions:

"What alternative is there to 'X' – are there any other options we could consider?"

"How might what you're suggesting affect me/my partner and our baby?"

"Would you please explain that a bit more as I don't understand fully?"

"Is my partner/baby OK?"

- and remember to use the BRAIN decision making tool.

Informed decision making makes for a positive birth! A woman and her partner who felt that they were able to ask relevant questions, get information and understand fully before agreeing to something will more likely feel empowered. This is such an important issue – it can potentially change the course of your experience during labour and birth, by how listened to and respected you feel during your birth, just by being fully involved and asking a few simple questions. During labour, you can ask for 5 minutes alone to think through what is being suggested, without someone hovering over you waiting for an immediate answer.

Chapter 12

Importance Of Breastfeeding

Breastfeeding comes with health benefits for both baby and mother. It is also a wonderful way for both mother and child to bond and understand each other in their own special way. You are now well prepared and know what to expect once you begin this wonderful breastfeeding journey.

We all want the best for our babies whether we choose to breastfeed or not. There are numerous breastfeeding benefits that you and your baby will enjoy.

For baby:

After birthing your baby, they will be place on your breast. Your baby will find her way to the nipple and begin suckling. This is the magical moment you have been waiting for, right? Baby will suckle for the very first time, and most importantly, get to partake of the nutritious Colostrum. Colostrum is the first milk which is thick and yellowish in colour. Colostrum is important for your baby because it contains a high concentration of antibodies and nutrients which your new born needs to start building a strong immune system.

Meconium is your baby's first poop. Colostrum helps your baby pass meconium because it contains laxative ability and results.

Breast milk contains a whole lot of vitamin and nutrient goodness that your baby needs to grow healthy and fight illnesses and infections. Just like building a house where we ensure that the foundation is strong, breastfeeding will also ensure a good start for your baby Health wise.

Breastfeeding creates quality bonding time for you and your baby. As your baby breastfeeds, they are able to register your smell and you as the mom, will recognise what every sound and cry from your baby means.

Benefits for Momma:

If you have breastfed before, do you remember the pain you felt in your abdomen while breastfeeding? That was your uterus contracting. Those contractions help in reducing the bleeding that continues after birth.

Breastfeeding can be a form of contraceptive, at least for the first six months after birth.

You gained a few or a lot of pounds while pregnant. Breastfeeding will help you reduce and/or eliminate the baby fat altogether.

Breastfeeding will eliminate the risk of engorgement since you will ensure that your baby has breastfed the accumulated milk.

As breastfeeding helps keep away infections and diseases from your baby's body, you will save on medical expenses since you will have few to almost no doctor's appointments, which is a very good thing, right?

To reap the full benefits of breastfeeding, please breastfeed your young one almost immediately or a few hours after birth, depending on when you and baby will be stable, up until 6 months. Simply put, breastfeed exclusively for 6 months.

Chapter 13

Post-Birth Responsibilities

One of the key lessons that will come in handy is to know the right way to talk to your kid. You have to be sure that you are following the details in an apt manner. Here, we are going to discuss the way you need to talk to your kid.

Your way of talking and the manner in which you get your points across is extremely important. It might not be easy to get your point across instantly, but when you keep trying, you will surely be able to explain to your kid the reason why you are so persistent on a specific topic.

So, let us talk about some of the key factors which you must keep in mind in order to ensure that your kid grows up to become a responsible adult.

The right grooming

When your child is growing up, you need to instill the right manners in them. If you are careful, you should face no difficulties in executing this step. The real trouble begins when the realization that you have ignored the grooming hits later in your life.

When you allow your child to choose his own way and you never really bothered to talk to him about important life lessons, it may not help much.

This is the reason: you will have to work on the kind of grooming you offer to your child.

When children are relatively young and naive, they are much more likely to follow whatever it is you tell them. So, instead of letting them go astray and realizing it a lot later in life, the smarter solution is to ensure that you are working on the specifics at the right age.

Here, I am going to share some of the best tips that will come in handy for you when you are looking to groom your child in an apt manner. Of course, this by no means infers that it is the complete list and you have to rigidly stick to it. Parenting, as mentioned before, is flexible work. You will never find any rules written in black and white. This book will be the guide that can show you the path, but the final execution is always upon you.

So, let me watch out for some really important points that are going to help you get a clear picture of how grooming and the way it is done is important early in their life.

Creating the right connection

In order to help your kid become a responsible adult, it is extremely important to make the right connection. Here are some top tips that can be handy.

Love conquers all

It doesn't take a genius to know that love has the power of conquering every possible frontier. When you love someone, it is very evident that they will like talking to you. It is hard to convince someone who has no love for you as compared to someone who loves you dearly. This is why you need to be sure that you love your child.

Some of us make the habit of being too stern or too strict when we are trying to make our kids responsible. But you need to know that lack of love can turn out to be an extremely troublesome point. When you want to ensure that you are doing a great job at parenting, nothing exceeds love.

You will have to give the right amount of love to your child because your inability to love will create a rift that nothing will be able to fill. This is why the main method to use is to first love your child and then look at every other aspect that can be of help.

Once you manage to win their trust and love, they are more likely to be receptive to all you have to say. Winning the hearts of children isn't a herculean task and here are a few points you need to know. No doubt, following these will be sure to fetch you good rewards and allow you to succeed in the aim of working things out.

Don't rebuke your child for every mistake they make.

When you want to discipline your child, you need to be sure you don't scold them every now and then. Ever wondered what rebuking would get you? Try and step in the shoes of your child and then judge whether or not you should choose to scold him or her. If you spend a lot of time rebuking your child, you will eventually end up losing their faith and trust and this can lead to a lot more trouble than what you had bargained for. There have been a lot of scientific researches and studies which have shown that scolding a child can have the wrong psychological repercussions on your children than what you might have been hoping for.

So, you need to know where to draw the line. I am not recommending you pamper your child to an extent that you entertain all their wishes, but in the end, be sure that you are not scolding them all the time either. This will break their inner confidence and it can even lead to resentment and dissatisfaction. This has the potential to permanently mar your relationship.

Let them get their point across

This is one important point a lot of people miss out on. If you find your child doing something wrong, you should not come to your own conclusions. Many times, it so happens that perspectives can really alter a situation. Coming to a hasty conclusion has a way of showing you the wrong picture. Even if your child is wrong, give him one chance to justify what he did. This opportunity for justification is one of the best ways of winning his confidence. It also sends out the right message to him: that every person deserves an explanation. And not just with parenting. We have seen a lot of relationships fall apart simply because people never let others justify what they did. This can be one of the major causes of splits. When you allow your child to put their point across, you are actually showing them how much you trust them. This is another psychological move as it will make your child once again see in the belief you have in them.

Show them the difference between right and wrong

When you grew up, you made a lot of mistakes, didn't you? This is why you need to sit down and explain your point as to why they shouldn't have done something. It is not going to be easy and you may need to explain it more times than what you had planned. But in the end it will be worth it. So, do not give up on the need to explain to your child what is right and the things they did wrong. When they are growing, they may get a wrong idea and in such cases, having the perfect mentor who is willing to teach them the different details is an ideal way of assessing where things went awry. Do not rush through parenting because it is something that you should love doing. When you are willing to be a part of your child's life, you will begin to cherish every single thing. When you are explaining the difference between right and wrong to your child, try and use as many examples as you possibly can. The imagination of a child is very vivid. When you can elaborate your ideas with the right stories, they are likely to follow it and will trust you as much as is possible for them. Once your child trusts you enough, they will believe your judgment and it will be easier to impart to them the right lessons.

These are the top three ways by which you can really love your little kid and make them grow into big adults who will one day make you proud of who they turned out to be. Of course you can add more to these points and you may come up with your own strategies and plans as well. The idea is to be sure you are following the key instincts and your children will love to spend time with you.

Modulate your tone

It is important to modulate your tone in a way that will help you improve the way your child connects with you. There are a lot of parents who lose their cool the moment their child is accused of doing something wrong. Do you really think shouting at the top of your voice is going to help matters? Isn't it a lot better to sit and talk it out rather than rebuke your child?

Children can detect even the slightest change in your tone and it can often send the wrong signal. When you wish for your children grow up to become responsible adults, scolding and using a harsh tone is not going to work. Rather you should make it a point to use an understanding tone.

Let them open up

When your tone comes across as harsh and haughty, it will make your children scared of you. Walk in their shoes and ask yourself would you ever like to confess something to someone you were scared of? The answer is, of course, not and so you need to be sure that you are trying the best way to explain your point without scaring your child.

If you want your kids to open up to you and accept where they have gone wrong, you first need to win over their trust. When your main aim is to allow your kids to become great adults, you need to make them understand the need and importance to own their mistakes.

Think of a situation wherein you came to know about the mistakes your child did. Of course it would hurt you and so wouldn't it be a lot better if your child came up to you and admitted the mistake himself or herself. While the focus should be on grooming your child in a way that they do not make any mistakes, it is important to note that it is human to make faults.

So, you should always have the kind of tone which will help you win the confidence and trust of your kids. We have seen parents who could evoke the right trust in their kids and this ensured that not only kids are skeptical of doing something wrong, but at the same time, they make sure to confide in their parents the moment they realize that they made a mistake.

Some of the key points which will turn out to be handy when you are looking to have a good tone are as follows.

Never get your pitch too loud. The moment you raise your voice louder than normal, it is sure to send the wrong message and this in turn is going to create a lot of troubles.

Don't wipe the concern from your tone. When you are talking to a child, remember you are addressing someone who is still young. When you remove the concern from your voice, they are likely to be scared and scaring someone is never the right way to teach a lesson.

Kindness can conquer the toughest of hearts. Once again, it is important that you are kind enough with your child. When you are kind to them, it will ensure that you will be able to put your opinion across and they are likely to listen to you too.

Speak softly but speak the facts. I do not believe in sugar coating facts. You need to state things the way they are. When you speak softly, it will allow you to teach your child the right way to talk. The lessons your children learn are the ones they see.

These are some of the points you must keep in mind. They will help you a great deal in ensuring that your kids will grow up to be responsible. Implementing all these points is not the easiest thing to do and you should be willing to understand every single aspect meticulously. It is only when you have actually understood these points that you will be able to improve your art of parenting in the best manner.

One more very important point you absolutely must remember all the time is not to shout at your child when you know that he/she is at fault. You have to first explain it clearly as to what they did wrong and how and where they went awry. Often children do not realize their mistakes and scolding them for something which was done unintentionally may hurt their confidence.

So, you should try and see their perspective, help them get a better and clear understanding and then work your way towards improving who they are and who they can turn out to be.

Conclusion

I hope this book has given you food for thought and faith in your incredible body and powerful mind. And I hope the suggested ideas for birth partners serve you well.

If you are being told 'you're not allowed to...' or 'you have to...' this is a sign that you need to ask questions! Always take the time to do your own research and ensure you are getting personalised care.

Whilst birth is unpredictable, there is so much you can do to make it positive even down to changing the labour ward room around.

Invest time and effort into practising the hypnobirthing and breathing techniques, starting daily practise as early as you can.

Consider an in depth antenatal course and/or a hypnobirthing course if you are open to this, attend a good pregnancy yoga class, work on your mindset by reading as much birth positivity as possible and block out all negativity.

Remember the BRAIN acronym – if you ask, there is usually always time for someone to take the time to explain things to you and possible another option available which hadn't been mentioned. You deserve clear explanations on the benefits and risks of things being offered to you, and being pointed to evidence that backs this up.

For the women reading this book - you were built to do this and you are truly amazing.

Baby Sleep Training

The No-Cry Newborn and Toddler Solutions to Teach your Child to Stop Crying, Sleep All Night and Boost Discipline. Step by Step Plan to Tired Parents and Improve their Daily Routine

Katharina Marie

Introduction

For starters, you must not forget where the children come from. More recently, the baby developed in very gentle conditions - inside the mother's womb. He knew neither hunger, nor thirst, nor cold, nor loud sounds, nor fatigue, nor daylight. He was never alone - his mother's movements kept him lulling him all the time. And now in front of him is the whole world that he has to open.

No one is talking about trying to repeat the conditions in the house in which the child was in her mother's tummy. He has already left here, and there is no turning back; he will have to adapt to his new habitat. However, it will be much easier for the baby to do this if we facilitate this transition.

We know how peaceful the child feels if mom or dad puts his head on his chest. We also know very well how irritated he reacts to loud noise or sudden movements. Take care that the child is comfortable, that he does not have to wait long when he wants to eat, watch his temperature - all this is part of the care that he needs.

Infants need help for a long period of time; they are unable to satisfy their own needs - both physical and emotional. Being next to the mother, the child gradually begins to discover for himself and his own body, its separation from the mother. Therefore, physical contact is very important, especially in the first months and years of life. The child feels protected and draws during those moments the courage he needs to move away from his parents, and calmly remain alone.

Most of the day, a newborn does sleep, on average, twenty hours—or at least sixteen to twenty hours. He often wakes up because he is hungry. Moments of vigor last for a short time, the child is almost always excited; he often cries. A very important point regarding the sleep of a newborn is that you must not forget that the baby falls asleep almost instantly with restless sleep.

Chapter 1

Learn Sleep Is Important

Sleep...it's something that we all need. It is critical for parents, babies, little children and well, everybody! Tragically, a considerable lot of us don't get enough of it - our babies included.

We, as a whole, need adequate amounts of sleep to function correctly, and it is especially significant in the advancement of these babies and youthful children. It is proven that sleep denied grown-ups experience issues focusing and performing and may suffer from mental and physical problems in the long haul. So, we can't expect a sleep-deprived baby to function either!

Sleep is fundamental for physical and mental revival, a functioning invulnerable framework, substantial development, and cognitive function. Without enough sleep, your baby will end up unstable, irritable, and sad. What's more, to exacerbate the situation, sleep-hardship in the early stages will further meddle with their more drawn out term limit with regards to profound, relaxing sleep.

Babies and children who don't get enough sleep are often unreasonably named 'fastidious' and 'unpredictable' when in actuality they are too depleted to even think about functioning correctly. It's a given that babies who suffer from this low quality of sleep often have parents who are likewise consumed and along these lines incapable of appreciating, caring for and sustaining their children as they might want.

As indicated by an ongoing report by the National Sleep Association, over 70% of newborn children and babies have a sleep problem.

If not treated, over half of babies who suffer from sleep problems will keep on encountering problems through pre-school and school-age.

An inadequate amount of sleep in babies and children is a threat to wellbeing, conduct, mindset, consideration, memory, and learning capacity.

A few parents feel that they have irritable, forlorn babies. "My baby cries throughout the day, whenever when he's awake...of COURSE he's difficult!" Fussy - yes. Incessantly irritable - no. A few babies might be more delicate and touchy. However, babies who are crying so much are doing as such, which is as it should be. Accepting there are no therapeutic inconveniences and that a baby isn't in torment, your baby might cry during the day because he's basically worn out! Regardless of whether he gets occasional cat naps to a great extent, it won't explain the general sleep hardship that is so vital to his prosperity.

So, first of all: If you figure your baby isn't getting the adequate amount of sleep to function correctly and be all around rested, it's an ideal opportunity to take care of business. Observe his everyday conduct and ask yourself a few questions:

How many naps does he take every day?

How long are these naps?

How long does he stay awake between naps?

How much sleep would he say he is getting during the evening?

In the wake of making sense of your baby's essential examples, you may need to reconfigure certain parts of his everyday sleep to guarantee your baby is well-rested and content

Why Baby Sleep Is So Important

Sleep...it's something that we all need. It is critical for parents, babies, little children and well, everybody! Tragically, a considerable lot of us don't get enough of it - our babies included.

We, as a whole, need adequate amounts of sleep to function correctly, and it is especially significant in the advancement of these babies and youthful children. It is proven that sleep denied grown-ups experience issues focusing and performing and may suffer from mental and physical problems in the long haul. So, we can't expect a sleep-deprived baby to function either!

Sleep is fundamental for physical and mental revival, a functioning invulnerable framework, substantial development, and cognitive function. Without enough sleep, your baby will end up unstable, irritable, and sad. What's more, to exacerbate the situation, sleep-hardship in the early stages will further meddle with their more drawn out term limit with regards to profound, relaxing sleep.

Babies and children who don't get enough sleep are often unreasonably named 'fastidious' and 'unpredictable' when in actuality they are too depleted to even think about functioning correctly. It's a given that babies who suffer from this low quality of sleep often have parents who are likewise consumed and along these lines incapable of appreciating, caring for and sustaining their children as they might want.

As indicated by an ongoing report by the National Sleep Association, over 70% of newborn children and babies have a sleep problem.

If not treated, over half of babies who suffer from sleep problems will keep on encountering problems through pre-school and school-age.

An inadequate amount of sleep in babies and children is a threat to wellbeing, conduct, mindset, consideration, memory, and learning capacity.

A few parents feel that they have irritable, forlorn babies. "My baby cries throughout the day, whenever when he's awake...of COURSE he's difficult!" Fussy - yes. Incessantly irritable - no. A few babies might be more delicate and touchy. However, babies who are crying so much are doing as such, which is as it should be. Accepting there are no therapeutic inconveniences and that a baby isn't in torment, your baby might cry during the day because he's basically worn out! Regardless of whether he gets occasional cat naps to a great extent, it won't explain the general sleep hardship that is so vital to his prosperity.

So, first of all: If you figure your baby isn't getting the adequate amount of sleep to function correctly and be all around rested, it's an ideal opportunity to take care of business. Observe his everyday conduct and ask yourself a few questions:

How many naps does he take every day?

How long are these naps?

How long does he stay awake between naps?

How much sleep would he say he is getting during the evening?

In the wake of making sense of your baby's essential examples, you may need to reconfigure certain parts of his everyday sleep to guarantee your baby is well-rested and content.

Sleep Training Your Baby

All individuals need to sleep. Sleeping is important because it gives the body a chance to recover and recharge. Grown-ups need 6 to 8 hours of sleep to unwind, while babies need a total of 8 hours of sleep at night and rest throughout the day. Sleeping has great significance in our lives, and it incorporates cell recovery and conditions the sensory system and in general aides in the development of our body, brain, and wellbeing. Babies need sleep to create muscles, skeletal structures, brain function, and different organs. Besides, sleep enables the body to regenerate fingernails, toenails, hair, and skin. Sleep animates your baby's development, and when this is accomplished, your baby can achieve a healthy life.

Choosing the Right Bed

It is recommended to set up a protected sleeping environment for your baby before he even comes home. You can buy a charming bunk and bed sheets from different stores. Baby retail outlet associates can inform you about the best bedding for your baby. To ensure your baby sleeps well, the bed or den must feel perfect. Your baby must have an agreeable bed and a quiet situation to advance rest.

The comfort of your baby's bed is only one concern. Another is that it ought to give security to them to get a good night sleep. The sheets ought to be agreeable and delicate for your baby's sensitive skin. A layer that is unpleasant or even too cushy lessens you baby's solace along these lines. It causes sleep interference. The bed ought to likewise be excellent for your baby's eyes. There is a wide range of brilliant plans and textures on the market today that makes choosing good quality bedding a fun and simple assignment for guardians.

Sleeping with Your Baby

The favorable fundamental position in sleeping with your baby is the expanded holding time. It is advantageous for you because it is anything but difficult to have your baby by your side, particularly when you are breastfeeding and being close is encouraging for your baby. As indicated by research, babies who sleep beside their moms have less problems sleeping and cry less. Co-sleeping gives your baby warmth, sound, aroma, contact, and other tactile input that causes your baby to react positively. Sleeping with your baby is exceptionally safe and gainful. Be that as it may, it depends on individual circumstances. If the guardians smoke or consume unlawful medications, sleeping with your baby is unsafe.

Not sleeping with your baby exposes him to potential dangers; for example, accidental. Besides, it is always ideal to use a firm but comfortable sleeping pad, and point of confinement the use of pad and covers. This could likewise be hard for your relationship because you may be close with your baby, however, less so with your partner since you might utilize the baby as a barrier between you and your partner. Sleeping with your baby requires specific precautionary measures to be taken to guarantee baby safety.

Sleep Baby Sleep

How frequently have you said this to your baby, yourself, and the universe? If just there was a magic answer to get baby to sleep. One that offered no mediation concerning a parent and was not at all problematic for the baby to learn.

That baby could be born with the sleep during that time quality that mysteriously kicks in when they are out of the belly. Sadly, that isn't the case. We do need to intercede, and it is an aptitude a baby must learn. Have you ever heard the phrase "sleep like a baby"? Well, I don't know about you, but, from what I've seen, relatively few kids sleep like a baby when they are born. Sure, they sleep during the day and for brief periods during the night, however more often than not they are sleeping when we could best deal with them being awake and awake when we could best deal with them being asleep.

The most widely recognized reason a baby won't sleep is that they don't know how. They can nod off on us, in the vehicle, with a soother, being shaken, and so on, yet can't stay asleep without our help. With the best intentions, we have created a situation where it is impossible for our baby to sleep as the night progresses. They need us to re-make the conditions under which they at first nodded off. We don't need to beat ourselves up over why we let this occur, but start learning why we need to make great baby sleep propensities.

Would it be a good idea for us to give our baby a chance to sob late into the night? It is impossible not to have some measure of crying when we execute baby sleep arrangements. There are a few techniques which tout no crying and that we ought not to enable our kid to cry at sleep time, but I have not observed these strategies to be robust, and I couldn't stay focused on them. Much research has been done on the mental part of permitting some crying during the sleep training process, and it indicates it was being innocuous and having no long-term effects. Our babies can communicate in one manner, and that is through crying. They are crying to voice their disappointment at the change, not out of inconvenience or broken-heartedness.

There is a step-by-step guide that will get you through new child sleep training with a negligible measure of crying and the capacity to remain with your baby until he nods off. You will be there to demonstrate to your baby you have not abandoned him but instead, are just cooperating with him in getting him to have legitimate sound sleep patterns for the remainder of his life.

No training plan is simple; you should submit yourself ultimately; however, realize that with persistence and tolerance, your baby will sleep during that time and during the day, as appropriate for his age. I have utilized this step by step myself and am thrilled with the outcomes. I have two cheerful, balanced, and rested youngsters and my significant other and I are thoroughly enjoying them consistently and are all able to sleep like a baby.

Baby Sleep Techniques

If you are another parent, you likely have been searching for baby sleep techniques to enable your infant to nap better at night. You are not the only one! Numerous inexperienced parents are experiencing sleep hardship, and this generally proceeds until the child is about a year old, sometimes more. By following these essential tips, you will make sure to see the dark circles under your eyes rapidly vanish, and you'll feel progressively invigorated and empowered in no time.

The most significant of all baby sleep techniques is to get your baby on a schedule as fast as could reasonably be expected, and unquestionably by about two months old. The general principle guideline is to follow the encouraging, changing, playtime and naptime pattern for the day so your infant becomes more acquainted with the daily practice and starts to learn what comes next in the process. Notwithstanding the daytime schedule, assemble a nighttime plan too. It could be as simple as a bath followed by a bottle, at that point you put your darling down in the bunk for the night. Follow similar advances every night, and the little one will bit by bit start to understand that after the bath comes a bottle, and after that, it is time for sleep.

Some baby sleep techniques will work for different babies; however, may not work for yours. Be that as it may, I suggest swaddling your baby before bed at any rate during the initial three months. It will, in general, work wonders for infants who need the coziness and comfort that they were used to in the belly. Continuously put your child to sleep on his or her back, per the American Association of Pediatrics' rules for averting sudden infant death syndrome or SIDS. They likewise suggest that babies utilize a pacifier at night as that appears to bring down the danger of SIDS also.

Ideally, these baby sleep techniques will enable you to get shut-eye progressively at night. What's more, if not, recollect that, they'll in the long run sleep as the night progresses - we as a whole figure out how to do it at some point!

Attempting to get your baby to rest at night can be a nightmare. For mothers and fathers, numerous sleepless nights have been spent trying to get their infants to fall into a sleeping pattern so they can get some rest. The awful truth is that baby sleep preparation can be both baffling and debilitating for the parent that has the obligation to get the baby to sleep. Getting your baby to sleep can be drawn nearer from multiple points of view, and baby sleep patterns are different from infant sleep patterns. It is safe to say that you are spending sleepless nights considering how to put your baby to sleep? Do you need a merited decent night's sleep? At that point, here are a few methods that can enable your baby to discover a pattern of sleep so you can get some rest.

Infant versus baby.

When you initially arrive home from the hospital with your new infant, you may see that the baby sleeps more often than not. Infants generally remain conscious for sustaining purposes, and the routine is unsurprising. Anyway, as they develop more, they spend more hours awake, and you will lose a great deal of sleep until you can get your baby acclimated to a sleeping pattern. This is when the parent will need to attempt intervention techniques to enable the baby to progress into a progressively adequate sleeping pattern. Intervention techniques do work, yet which one you choose depends on your individual circumstances.

The Ferber method.

Utilizing the Ferber method implies that when your baby is alert, however, prepared to rest, the baby is put to bed, and the parent leaves the room. If the baby cries, the parent does not return to the space for five minutes. Whenever when the baby cries out once more, the parent will wait ten minutes to respond. This process is repeated, including additional time between the interims when the parent returns to reassure the crying youngster until they fall asleep. On a subsequent night, the parent will include the additional time the main event and increment the time that they return until in the end, and the baby figures out how to sleep alone.

The steady parent removal method.

The steady parent removal method includes remaining with your baby after you put them to bed. The parent will sit near the den until the baby falls asleep for two nights. On the third and fourth nights, the parent will sit farther away from the bed until the baby falls asleep once more. This process is repeated until the parent is no longer in the room, and the baby has figured out how to sleep without anyone else's presence.

The cry out method.

With the cry out method, the arrangement is a straightforward one, put the baby to bed and give them a chance to cry themselves to sleep. This method can test the desire of any minding parent who needs to sit idle while their kid cries out for a long time.

TODDLER SLEEP TRAINING TECHNIQUES

Avoiding Trouble Spots

I believe it is the parents' business to provide the right environment when their toddler rests. Bedtime is not a good time to holler at your child or partner, have long telephone conversations, or fail to give your toddler the attention he needs. Not many children sleep well if they feel tense, miserable, or dismissed.

Right off the bat, help your child feel that her bed is someplace she can go to feel safe. Parents can help make a bed a cheerful spot by putting a couple of favorite plush toys and a darling cover on it. Try not to utilize the crib or bed as a punishment. Your toddler will not have affectionate associations with her bed if you send her there when she is "being bad."

Be that as it may, by a long shot, the most important way a parent can help a toddler is by letting him figure out how to fall asleep alone. For instance, if you have consistently rocked your child to sleep, have a go at holding him, patting him gradually, and after that putting him down when his eyes are still open.

If you have consistently given your daughter a chance to fall asleep with the bottle, take a stab at giving her a bottle in a dim room and after that putting her to bed without the bottle before she falls asleep. Says one dad: "Our daughter was so used to sleeping with the bottle that if she woke up at all in the night, she would instantly yell out, 'Bottle.' At one point she was having four bottles per night! She had no clue how to fall asleep without one."

Not surprisingly, first-time parents, for the most part, have the most issues with sleep. It can be so difficult to leave a little, cuddly child alone in obscurity. "There was not any more magnificent sensation than feeling that tiny infant when I held her in my arms and rocked her to sleep," says one mother. In any case, as time goes on, most parents never again feel so sentimental about night time closeness.

Afterward, from the same mother: "My daughter never again feels so great in my arms since I'm worn out! In addition to the fact that I have to rock this thirty-pound child for one hour at night, yet if she awakens, I need to do it again and again." This parent had reached her limits. Within a week, she had begun a campaign to get her daughter to fall sleep in her crib.

The Effects of Sleep Training

With baby sleep training experts, specialists and guardians all offering guidance on getting your baby to sleep with hot features, for example, make your baby sleep from 7pm-7am, it is no big surprise numerous people are tuning in. This training conflicts with our senses and as you may have seen feels appalling to endure. I accept these beginnings in life are the most critical, and sleep training is jeopardizing close bonds, connections, and trust.

When a baby cries, it is calling for attention. Crying shows that the baby is uncomfortable (wet, hot, cold), hungry, in pain, scared or tired. A normal response in people is to react to this crying to ensure we address that need. It is the reason we cannot stand a baby crying and why there is an inclination to help. A baby will weep for these reasons. If you take care of these problems, they will quit crying.

Overtired - Rock them off to sleep in your arms in a dark room.

Wet Diaper/Nappy

Cold or Hot

Wind Pain

Getting teeth

Cerebral pain, Fever or Illness

Not all problems above can be addressed rapidly; however, ameliorating them in some way will help, or you might probably get something to mitigate them. Likewise paying little respect to whether you changed a diaper, check once more! A baby comes into this world, realizing that it has a mother and close family (counting father) to take care of and care for it. It doesn't know much else about the world as it has a lot to gain from you. So, when they are set in a quiet, dark room and are either scared or uncomfortable and they shouted out for assistance, and no one came. They continued crying to an ever-increasing extent, and still, no one came. What does this tell them?

That when they are separated from everyone else and scared or need assistance, nobody is there for them and they are alone in this world. When you see a world of people not caring about others, do you figure it may have originated from others not caring about them when they were first born? So, when your baby is crying, comfort them, go in and ensure they are alright. It will mean getting up in the middle of the night, yet in the long haul, they will self-settle more easily and be a progressively sure tyke realizing that if they do need assistance, you are there.

Baby Sleeping Tips And Requirements

Rest is imperative to children's wellbeing and development. If your baby does not get enough rest, he may experience difficulty getting through the day and particularly the night. As a parent, it is excellent to realize that napping encourages a baby to rest adequately at night, so it is an off-base conviction that keeping your baby awake during the daytime will make him rest better at night.

Getting baby to rest might be a difficult time for most parents. Most parents look forward to the night they can put their baby to rest in the nursery and get some undisturbed rest for themselves. If the baby frequently wakes up during the night, the parents get effectively depleted as well. Along these lines, it is fundamental to defeat your baby's sleeping issues when you can to help your baby achieve wellbeing and development. Getting your baby to rest isn't a simple occupation and extensive baby rest preparing is required.

Infants

Infants regularly rest at least sixteen hours every day. As your baby's sensory system develops, he will build up a progressively predictable sleep pattern later in his life. Be that as it may, at 3 months, numerous infants rest for about five hours at a time. Furthermore, by 6 months, their resting hours are inside nine to twelve hours.

3 To 6 Months

At 3 months, the baby's resting propensities will turn out to be increasingly reliable. As of now, you can start building up an ordinary nap plan. Infants have their very own comprehension, and they need the correct signs to know when the time has come to rest. Regardless of whether it doesn't work quickly, soon your baby will begin to learn it. By four months, babies need, at any rate, three naps every day; in the first part of the day, evening, and early at night.

6 Months To 1 Year

During this time of your baby's life, the average rest is fourteen hours per day, yet anything less or more can be typical for your baby. Children's nap times change from 3 naps every day to 2; longer naps in the first part of the day and toward the evening.

Baby Sleeping Tips

Put your baby to bed when he is sleepy yet wakeful utilizing an agreeable, level, and delicate bedding. A pacifier may likewise assist your baby with sleeping comfortably; however, never use this until breastfeeding is entrenched. Try not to put your baby in bed with a bottle on his side. A predictable daytime and nighttime rest schedule is useful, and keeping up a steady bedtime routine is necessary.

You can likewise utilize baby tranquilizers to assist your baby with sleeping. The important thing is a delicate cover which does keep your baby comfortable and provides security and warmth. Music can likewise be useful, and you can play your baby's preferred bedtime song to quiet him and make his relaxing time more pleasant.

Furthermore, babies under six months ought not to rest in the same bed as their parents because studies show an increased danger of Sudden Infant Death Syndrome (SIDS). Around 50% of infants who die of SIDS are in a bed-imparting to their parents' circumstance. Factually, one in every 2,000 infants dies of SIDS every year.

Chapter 2

Learn Newborns Sleep Patterns

A sleeping baby seems very active to an outside observer. He moves his eyes—sometimes, even lifting his eyelids. Sometimes, he begins to move his arms and legs. He can begin to make quiet sounds, even cry a little.

However, the impression is misleading - the child is actually sleeping. He even dreams. But his dream is very superficial, and the baby is easy to wake up with noise or movements. This is definitely not the best moment to take care of a child, mistakenly believing that he needs your help.

If the child continues to sleep, he will go to a restful sleep. For three hours of continuous sleep, the child goes from two to three cycles of restless and calm sleep. Each of them will account for approximately 50 percent of the total sleep time.

A newborn, when he sleeps or is awake, absolutely does not distinguish between day and night. It must be fed and taken care of around the clock. He has no control over his sleep or his needs. This is debilitating but only temporary. Do not be surprised if your child's sleep during this period is a little chaotic and unpredictable.

The task of parents in the first few weeks of a child's life is to get to know their baby and to give them the opportunity to get to know them. Parents discover, trying not to interfere in this process, at what moments the child falls asleep, in what position he likes to sleep, does he like to be swung smoothly or more rhythmically, etc. They learn to understand his cry and respond to the needs that they can determine, not forgetting that every week, it will make it easier and simpler, as the child learns to express them better.

The difficulties that parents do face are very often associated with their own fatigue. They have to endure a painful awakening due to crying and sleepless nights. A few weeks are enough to exhaust them to oblivion.

Adapting to your child, learn to adapt to his rhythm, that is, relax in those moments when he sleeps.

Getting used to having a newborn baby can be difficult for parents. The biggest change for most parents can be getting acclimated with baby sleep patterns. It is an indisputable fact that new parents can expect numerous sleepless nights, so understanding what kind of sleep their baby will get might help parents to acknowledge what these initial couple of months will look like.

A newborn baby, generally, does little more than sleep and eat. This keeps mother occupied with breastfeeding and nonstop diaper changes. Baby sleep patterns for the initial three weeks ought to be an aggregate of 16-20 hours of sleep each day. Since they will sleep for around 2 hours at a time, this means parents may almost certainly take short naps for the initial three weeks or should sleep in shifts. At three weeks, the baby will start sleeping 16 to 18 hours a day, maybe sleeping for more extended periods. At six weeks, the baby will sleep even less, around 15 to 16 hours a day. This means parents could expect to sleep a little more at this age.

The age of four months means the baby will sleep 9 to 12 hours at night in addition to 2 naps during the day. Parents will cheer as baby sleep patterns, at last, enable them to get an entire night's sleep. Throughout the following couple of months, the baby will keep on having increasingly stable sleep patterns and offer parents a truly necessary break from interfering with sleep. These baby sleep patterns are fundamental for baby to get the nourishment and solace she needs to grow properly. Trying to understand what's in store at different stages can help set up the unseasoned parents for the sleep they will almost certainly get as a baby develops.

Chapter 3

Study The Stages Of Sleep And Sleep Cycles

Babies require more sleep compared to adults, especially when they are very young. The average baby less than 3 months old tends to sleep twice as much as his or her parents, with half of this sleeping period occurring in the daytime. You may have noticed your child waking up frequently especially during the day. This is because babies do not sleep in one long stretch; they need to wake up for regular feedings.

While all newborns sleep a majority of the day, no two babies have the exact same sleep cycle. Generally, however, the average infant can be expected to sleep in intervals of about 2 hours each during the day and from 4 to 6 hours at nighttime.

What are the phases of sleep? Babies go through different phases of sleep just as adults do. Although you may not be aware of it and think sleep is as simple as closing your eyes and then waking up the next day, there are actually different stages of sleep that you go through. In addition, there are levels of sleep that you cycle through, going from drowsiness to light sleep to dream sleep and then to deep sleep. The dream sleep cycle is also referred to as rapid eye movement or REM sleep. The cycle continues until you eventually wake up, with adults going through the process on average five times a night.

The same process holds true for babies. In fact, your baby began experiencing sleep cycles even before birth. He or she would already have gone through dream sleep even while in your uterus, at about 6 or 7 months of gestation.

You can determine whether your baby is undergoing dream sleep or non-dream sleep by observing him or her while resting. When the infant is undergoing REM or dream sleep, you will note the eyes darting back and forth under the eyelids, the breathing becoming irregular, and the body remaining quite still, save for a few twitches now and then.

When your baby is in a non-dream sleep, also called quiet sleep, breathing will be regular and deep, and he or she may also emit an occasional big sigh. During this period, the baby will be lying very still but the mouth may be making small sucking movements or the whole body can give a sudden start. These sudden start movements are also called "hypnagogic startles" and are considered normal occurrences for babies.

These "hypnagogic startles" happen to adults and older children too. They occur most often when you are just about to fall asleep. This non-dream sleep is well developed in newborns. However, they occur in short little bursts as compared with the continuous flow that adults and older children experience. This pattern will be increasingly continuous for your newborn during the first month of life until the startles gradually disappear.

When babies hit 3 months, they will gradually begin sleeping more through the night and less during the daytime. The average 3-month old baby sleeps twice as long during the night than during the day. By the time babies reach 6 months old, daytime naps will grow gradually longer, but fewer naps will be required. At that age, your baby may only be taking two naps during the day at a length of 1 to 2 hours each. At the same time, most babies will be clocking in an average of 12 hours each night. However, you can still expect the odd arousals in between.

When your baby is 1 year old, he or she may be sleeping a total of 12 to 14 hours in total, which includes a daytime nap (usually just one at this point). When your baby reaches 2 years old, this nap may or may not be dropped.

In order to start instilling good sleeping habits, you can practice managing your baby's naps. It is a wonderful idea not to let your little one nap too late in the day as this may interfere with sleep later on in the evening. Chances are, the later the nap is in the day, the later the bedtime at night, as your child may not need to doze off so soon after a nap.

You are advised instead to isolate naps to the earlier parts of the morning and afternoon. On getting a little older, it is recommended that the main nap be a little after lunch, making certain that there is a wide gap between waking up and going to bed at night. Some believe that it is essential for your child to have an appropriate amount of new experiences to "file away" at night, as dreams.

Like a regular adult, the sleep-wake cycle of your baby directly relates to the rhythm of body temperature, feeding, and hormone release. These things greatly influence the biological cycle (also called circadian rhythm), through which bodies pass during 24-hour intervals. Human beings fall asleep when their adrenal hormone levels drop along with their temperatures and then wake up as body temperatures and hormonal levels rise again.

Keep in mind that it may be more difficult to fall asleep when hormone and body temperature levels are high. It is also more difficult to wake up when these factors are low. This explains why travelers experience jet lag and shift workers have to adjust to their graveyard shifts or unusual hours in order to function well.

Some people are naturally better at staying up or getting up late at night, which is why some parents are more tolerant and welcoming of their baby waking them up at night as well.

Baby's Sleep Stages

Newborns (1 to 3 months)

It is not a good idea to start sleep training a newborn. Not only are they not physically and emotionally mature enough to handle sleep training, they also need to feed on milk every few hours or so. Employing sleep training techniques on a newborn will interfere with their feeding, which means they may not get enough of their required nutrients for the day.

What you can do to help a newborn acquire good sleeping habits is provide exposure to natural light. This practice helps set your baby's circadian rhythm early on in life and helps to avoid sleep problems later on. Your circadian rhythm is also known as your body clock.

You have probably observed your sleeping newborn and have noticed something like a startled motion affecting the whole body. This is also called "moro" reflex, which may or may not cause the baby to wake up. Some babies may go back to sleep while others may get disturbed or angry and may need to be soothed back to sleep.

Once your baby has reached 6 weeks, you can start establishing a bedtime routine which will promote an expectation of sleep and to some extent set the infant's body clock. As the parent, you can pretty much decide for yourself what to include in this bedtime routine. Some good activities include giving a warm sponge bath, singing a lullaby, dancing or swaying your child to sleep, reading a bedtime story, or providing one last feeding before tucking your little one in.

Around this same time, you can also start introducing a set time for when your baby should go to sleep. Be sure to stick to that schedule as closely as you can; this is essential to your sleep training. Of course, there may be some exceptions which require you, as a parent, to exercise wisdom and discretion, such as when the child is sick or when you are traveling.

Just the same, you must also start waking your little one up at the same time each morning. This includes naps as well. Make it a habit to lay your child down for naps at the same time each morning and afternoon. Doing so sets the stage for sleep training and before long, your little one will come to expect these napping, bed, and waking up times.

You can adjust these sleeping routines and schedules as you see fit. It won't take long before your baby starts to mature, needs fewer naps in the daytime, and sleeps more during the night. Be aware and modify the routine accordingly.

3 to 6 months

Around 4 months old, you will start to notice your baby having a more developed sense of sleep and wake patterns. It may delight you to know that fewer nighttime feedings will be necessary. That means more sleep for you!

However, you still need to exercise caution; even if your baby is showing (some) signs of independence, it does not mean that you can suddenly impose a strict sleep regimen. Remember, you are still dealing with a baby, so be mindful of this fact.

Perhaps your little one is already showing good sleeping patterns that fit quite well into your present family life. Maybe you do not need to employ sleep training at all. However, if you still feel that your baby is not getting enough sleep and would like him or her to sleep longer, 4 to 5 months is the best time for you to impose some kind of a sleep training regimen.

It is important for you to observe your child's response to your sleep training. If the infant doesn't seem to be handling it well or doesn't appear ready for it yet, then there is no need to be strict. Take a step back and slow down. You can always try again in a couple of weeks.

Even if things seem to be progressing well, there may come a time when your baby suddenly starts waking up again in the middle of the night. This can be confusing or even frustrating, especially after you finally started getting your sleep back on track. Don't worry. Even when babies have been sleeping through the night for weeks or even months, it's very normal for them to suddenly start waking up again in the middle of the night.

Aside from training your baby to stay asleep, another important element of sleep training is getting him or her to fall asleep without assistance. If your baby is unable to fall asleep independently, you will have to teach him or her how to. It's an essential skill babies need to master to get the most out of their sleep. One method to help move the process along is to begin putting your child down in the crib when sleepy but still awake.

If your baby doesn't sleep right away and you think additional assistance is needed, you can begin trying out more involved techniques of sleep training. Other methods are available, such as the CIO and the "No Cry" methods. Remember that your parenting style, your values and beliefs, as well as your child's personality are what will help you decide on the best kind of training method to use.

6 to 9 months

Once babies reach 6 months, they will be able to divide up to 14 hours of sleep into nighttime sleep and daytime naps. It may delight you to know that your baby is now capable of sleeping for much longer stretches of time.

Around 6 to 9 months, babies may begin to consolidate daytime sleep into a number of naps. Their schedule may look something like this: one nap in the morning, another one in the afternoon, and one last one early in the evening. If your little one seems to need more than just three naps a day, do not be concerned, as this is perfectly normal. What is important is that you keep consistent time schedules for both naps and bedtime. Again, this is crucial in regulating sleep patterns.

How many hours of sleep a night is your baby getting now? If your answer is a good 9 or 10 hours a night, it's a good sign that your little one has learned how to go back to sleep independently; otherwise, he or she would still be crying and looking for you or some other form of soothing. If you find yourself able to sleep just as well, then congratulations! You have been raising a good sleeper.

Now this age is also perfect to wean your baby from night feeding, if this is what you prefer. However, be sure to observe your baby's reaction to night weaning. Most babies should be ready for it by now, but if your child does not respond well to it, then slow down and try again in a few weeks. There is certainly no reason to rush your baby to do something he or she is not yet ready for.

Again, your baby may have other reasons for waking up other than wanting to feed. Remember, we all wake up at night for short spells, whether as toddlers or adults. While adults have the capabilities to get back to sleeping immediately, your baby may not understand how to self-soothe yet and may wake you up crying. This doesn't necessarily mean he or she wants to nurse.

There is no need to worry when your baby starts to wake up again at night and have difficulty going back to sleep. This is very normal for babies aged 9 months all the way up to 1 year.

There are, in fact, several reasons for this. First, your child may wake due to teething discomfort. Second, your toddler may experience separation anxiety, prompting these wake-up calls. Separation anxiety is pretty normal for babies at this age. Your baby is increasingly becoming aware of you at this age and may want to be with you at all times. Waking up and realizing there is no one else in the room may result in some distress, which often eases once you enter the room and offer a greeting.

In addition, from 6 months all the way up to 1 year, babies are absorbing and learning a lot of new skills. They may be in the process of figuring out how to sit up on their own, crawl, and even stand up and walk on their own. Indeed, this time is filled with exciting, new developments for your little baby. Your baby may be so pumped up about these new skills that he or she may even be trying them out during sleep! Believe it or not, your baby may actually just try to sit up and wake in the process.

As for establishing healthy sleeping habits for your baby at this age, it is pretty much the same as when your baby was 3 to 6 months old. To recap, sleep training refers to the practice of developing a bedtime pattern. Whether it's a warm bath, a lullaby, a bedtime tale or a cuddle—always do things in a similar order. These activities will help set the stage for your baby's sleep.

Come up with a consistent routine for your baby. This does not mean your baby gets lunch at the exact same time each day. You just need to formulate a predictable daily schedule that helps your baby to fall asleep at nearly the same time.

Encourage the child to sleep without your assistance. Again, simply lay your baby down in the crib when drowsy but still wide awake and have a plan in place in the event he or she cries once you leave the room. Try letting some minutes pass to establish whether your little one is really upset or just fussing a little before buckling down to sleep.

If your baby fusses a lot when laid in the crib, try setting bedtime thirty minutes earlier. It could just be that your baby is overtired, making it harder to settle down. An earlier bedtime may help him or her sleep better at night.

Chapter 4

Create A Sleep Friendly Space

Your loved ones may not hold back on giving their "best" advice to help you and your little one get a good night's sleep. However, even though they mean well, it is sometimes frustrating to get one piece of advice after another that sometimes don't make sense.

So in this chapter, I have listed some healthy sleep practices from experts and parents to help you decide which one works for your child.

Place your baby in the "best" sleep position – There are some infants who find it more comfortable to sleep on their tummies or on their sides. My firstborn, Ethan, for example, slept better when he was placed on his tummy, but then we learned that this position is dangerous for infants.

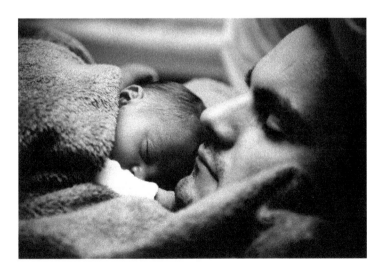

In fact, according to pediatricians, babies who sleep on their sides or on their tummies are at a higher risk of **SIDS or Sudden Infant Death Syndrome**. The American Academy of Pediatrics (AAP) recommends that the best sleep position for babies up to 1-year-old is on their backs.

- **Be sensitive to your baby's cues** – Make sure that your baby is comfortable and full. The key here is to keep an eye on your little one's cues. Meet his/her needs first so that he is content and comfortable before putting him to sleep.

- **Consider the time of putting your baby to sleep** – Set a schedule of when you will put your baby to sleep and make sure that you stick to this time. Your baby will more likely adapt to this and will become sleepy at this hour after a few weeks.

While nap time is important, you don't want your baby to take a nap that is too close to his/her usual nighttime sleeping schedule.

- **Create a sleep-friendly environment** – This is one of the tips that I found most effective for my son. Since newborns do not know what day and night are, you can start teaching them this concept by doing the following:

In the daytime, put your baby down to nap in rooms that are not too quiet because you want him/her to recognize that there are plenty of (noisy) activities at that time of the day.

At night, make sure that you keep the sounds to a minimum, and put away anything that can stimulate your child. Keep the lights low and use only your soft voice when speaking to him/her.

Make sure that the room temperature is comfortable so that your baby won't overheat or be too cold. Babies are at a higher risk of SIDS when they get too hot. A good room temperature is somewhere around 16-20 °C (60-70 °F).

- **Use swaddles** – Most infants sleep soundly at night when they are swaddled **properly**. Swaddling makes newborns feel like they are safe and sound in their mother's womb.

  Younger babies also often experience startle reflex (or Moro reflex) that can wake them up. This is reduced when babies are swaddled. Swaddling has also been seen to help reduce the risk of *SIDS*. Keep in mind, however, that you should stop swaddling when your baby has learned to roll over.
- **Begin to practice a pre-bedtime routine** – It's never too early to begin a pre-sleeping routine. This will give your little one a cue that bedtime is soon coming. You could include things like giving him/her a sponge bath, reading a book, or dimming the lights.

What is SIDS?

The National Institute of Child Health and Human Development defines SIDS as "a sudden and silent medical disorder that can happen to an infant who seems healthy." A report from the AAP shows that SIDS is the leading cause of fatalities beyond the newborn stage and can also occur anytime until the child is a year old.

SIDS is also referred to as "crib death" because it is associated with the time when the baby is sleeping. There are many things that parents can do to reduce the risk of SIDS, some of which are:

- Always place your little one to sleep on his/her back.

- Only place your baby on a firm or flat surface. Use only a fitted sheet—avoid any loose items in his/her crib.

- Breastfeeding is proven to help reduce SIDS by 50%.

- Consider sharing your room with your baby at least in his/her first 6 months, and place his/her bed close to yours.

- Never put toys, crib bumpers, pillows or blankets in your baby's sleeping area.

- Make sure that your baby wears proper sleeping attire to keep his/her body at the right temperature.

- Consider giving your child a Soothie or pacifier as it can actually reduce the risk of SIDS. If you're exclusively breastfeeding, you want to make sure that you establish breast-feeding your child first before offering a pacifier as otherwise it could cause nipple confusion.

- If you're still expecting, make sure you stop smoking and avoid being around with people who smoke. The risk of SIDS increases for moms who smoked during their pregnancy.

The healthy sleep practices that were discussed in this chapter are great ideas to start with. Keep in mind that it may take time and some trial and error before you can achieve the results you want.

Chapter 5

Establish A Routine

Establishing a routine will help create some predictability in your day. It helps your baby know when certain things are going to happen. A predictable routine decreases anxiety about what's to come, and the end result is a more complaisant baby, especially when it's sleepy time. A typical routine would include feedings in line with your pediatrician's recommended feeding times, some regular fun play or activity time, and then, of course, sleep time, based on your baby's natural rhythm dictating when they need to sleep.

Eat, play, sleep

No matter your baby's age, she is in a repetitive cycle of eating, playing, and sleeping throughout the day. Ideally, you want to keep the activities in this order to prevent a feed-to-sleep association, in which a baby expects to be fed right before she goes to sleep. A baby who is fed to sleep typically wakes in between sleep cycles and asks to be fed *back* to sleep. Separating the feeding and sleep with an activity is a smart start to teaching good sleep habits.

Here's a sample of what an eat, play, sleep schedule might look like for a six-month-old:

» 7:00: Awake for the day

» 7:30: Eat

» 8:00–9:00: Play

» 9:30–10:30: Nap 1

» 10:45: Eat

» 11:15 a.m.–12:30 p.m.: Play

» 1:00–2:00: Nap 2

» 2:15: Eat

» 2:45–4:00: Play

» 4:30–5:15: Sleep (catnap)

»5:30: Eat

»5:45–6:45: Play

»7:00: Eat

»7:15: Bedtime routine

»7:45: Asleep

Please follow your pediatrician's recommendations for feeding schedules.

QUICK FIX If your baby is waking prematurely from sleep, such as always taking short naps or waking too early in the morning, you may want to add a short activity between waking up and eating: eat, play, sleep, play, then repeat. This will further dissociate feeding from sleep. If baby is waking too early, he may be doing so because he knows that the moment he wakes, he will get his favorite thing in the world: a feeding. But if your baby knows that he will have to do something else first when he wakes, this will encourage him to go back to sleep if he wakes up too early.

Recognize drowsy signs

It's important to learn your baby's tiredness signs, so you don't miss her sleepy window: that prime window of opportunity to put your baby down for bed. Putting a baby down to sleep when she's over- or under-tired can result in a teary struggle. The sweet spot for putting your baby down is when she is just starting to get tired, but before she gets overtired. When a baby gets overtired, her body compensates by producing adrenaline. She ends up wired, rather than tired.

Here are some typical sleepy cues:

» Eye rubbing

» **Yawning**

» **Fussiness**

» Noises/yelling, or cries that gradually increase in length and frequency

» Decrease in activity

» Loss of interest in playing

set bedtime and wake-up time

Want to set your baby's internal clock? Keep a set bedtime and wake-up time. When a baby goes to sleep and wakes up at about the same times each day, his body starts to produce certain hormones at those times to aid sleep, and wake him up when it's time to get up. This is part of your baby's internal biological clock.

Putting a baby to sleep at 6:30 p.m. one night, and 9:00 p.m. the next night, for example, not only disrupts her internal clock but also makes it very difficult for her to fall asleep and stay asleep. Keeping a consistent bedtime and wake-up time is an important component of improving your baby's sleep.

AGE	NUMBER OF NAPS	NAP SLEEP	NIGHT SLEEP	TOTAL SLEEP
NEWBORN	Several	5–8 hours	Varies	14–17 hours
3 MONTHS	4	2–4 hours	10–12 hours	14–17 hours

6 MONTHS	2–3	2–3.5 hours	10–12 hours	12–15 hours
9 MONTHS	2	2–3 hours	10–12 hours	12–15 hours
12 MONTHS	1–2	2–3 hours	10–12 hours	11–14 hours
18 MONTHS	1	2–3 hours	10–12 hours	11–14 hours
24 MONTHS	0–1	0–2 hours	10–12 hours	11–14 hours

That said, you don't have to obsess over keeping the bedtime exact each night. Up to a 30-minute difference rarely has any impact on sleep. And if your baby occasionally wants to sleep in, like on a cozy Sunday morning, let him! You can adjust by shortening one of his naps.

An ideal bedtime for babies over 3 months old up to toddlerhood is between 7:00 p.m. and 8:30 p.m. An ideal wake-up time is between 6:00 a.m. and 8:30 a.m. Of course, individual variations in schedule may be necessary due to work or other commitments. These are suggested bedtimes and wake-up times in an ideal world. We all know that ideal is not always possible, and that's fine. Follow these times if they work for you, and if you can't, just adjust to your family's schedule.

Newborns don't really follow set bedtimes and wake-up times, since they have immature and underdeveloped internal clocks. Their bedtime tends to be late, since they have a hard time settling for bed in the early evening. This is a phenomenon known as the "witching hour." It is not unusual for newborns to settle after 9:00 or 10:00 p.m., and sometimes even later. Don't stress, and don't try to force your newborn to fall asleep early; just follow her lead. Over time, you'll notice that your baby will start to accept an earlier bedtime. Somewhere between three and four months of age, your baby should settle into a bedtime of around 8:00 or 8:30 p.m.

Create a bedtime routine

Bedtime routines are a wonderful opportunity for both you and your baby to relax, unwind, and bond. They are also important signals to your baby that bedtime is coming. When your baby knows what's coming, she will be much less apprehensive. Some babies even look forward to the bedtime routine. Here are some things to keep in mind when creating a bedtime routine:

Have Fun! Your routine should be enjoyable for both you and your baby. Include things like lullabies, bedtime books, cuddling, or anything else both you and your baby enjoy.

Not Too Short, Not Too Long. With a short routine, your baby won't have enough time to unwind. A routine that is too long may disinterest your baby. An ideal routine is 20 to 25 minutes long, or 10 to 15 minutes for a newborn up to three months old.

Keep It Simple. I always tell parents that the routine should be simple enough that when you are not home for bedtime, you can still implement some of the activities to help cue your baby to sleep. If your bedtime routine is very elaborate, it may be hard to replicate it on the go. This may discourage you from going out, and you deserve an occasional night out past bedtime!

Keep Bath Time Separate From The Bedtime Routine. I typically don't consider bath time a part of the bedtime routine. For one, most babies don't need a bath every single night. Bathing your baby every night just for the sake of routine is not very practical, and you will drive yourself nuts trying to implement this every night! You should have a sufficient routine (20 to 25 minutes) that does not include bathing. Second, consider the times when you are out at dinner or a friend's house, and can't give your baby a bath. As above, keep it simple for success!

EXTRA HELP: GOING OUT

You *can* go out and stay out past bedtime. Making sure you are home at 7:00 p.m. every night will put a huge strain on your social life, and you just don't need to be that firm. Your baby will be fine if she stays up past her bedtime occasionally, or falls asleep in the car on the way home. If you know that you'll be out late, bring your baby's pjs, make sure she has her last feeding, use a key phrase to cue sleep, such as "it's sleepy time," and lay her down anywhere you are. When you get home, just transfer your baby to the crib; no need to go through the bedtime routine again.

Chapter 6

Handle Night Wakings

Your baby is asleep! But now what? Perhaps you are anxiously waiting for her to wake up screaming. The first few nights she may just do this to see if you're really serious about this whole independent sleep thing. To keep things consistent, you will want to handle the night wakings in a very similar way to bedtime. Here's what you need to know.

When to stay away

When your baby wakes, it is very important to give her enough time to figure out how to fall asleep without your help. Delaying your intervention is the single most important part of nipping night wakings in the bud. Often, if given enough time, a baby will fall back asleep on her own. Once she does that, her sleep will typically improve dramatically, even to the point of sleeping through the night shortly thereafter.

How long you wait before you intervene depends on many factors, but it should be at least three to five minutes. This is how long it takes a baby to fully awaken and even realize she's awake. Intervening before this time may actually fully awaken your baby, and at that point it will be difficult for her to go back to sleep. Giving your baby enough time will help you confirm she is fully awake, and not just transitioning in between sleep cycles.

166

It's not unusual for a baby who is first learning to sleep independently to cry out in his sleep, and then drift back to sleep. Waiting to intervene also gives your baby a fair chance to practice going back to sleep on his own. Now, you are probably thinking: "You want me to wait until my baby completely wakes up before going to him?" Yes, absolutely! Remember we are working on independent sleep, meaning we want your baby to fall asleep on his own at bedtime and subsequently during the night. We are no longer "maintaining"; we are full-on working to teach your baby to sleep on his own. This means if he wakes, we want him to go back to sleep unassisted.

Going in too early is the number-one mistake parents make during night wakings. I totally understand this—I've done it myself! You want to quickly run in there before your baby fully wakes so everyone can just drift back to sleep. But this is often what starts the sleep troubles in the first place. Your baby has not learned how to transition in between sleep cycles on her own and keeps waking and expecting you to do it for her. If you keep fearing that your baby will wake, scream, and not go back to sleep, these wakings will just continue. Now is the time to work on this. Be strong—you've got this!

Safety Check

✓ When waiting to intervene, please make sure that you can see or hear your baby (for example, on a video monitor), and you know that there isn't anything wrong. The crib should be safe, and if safety is a concern, please check on your baby first.

✓ Your baby's needs should always be met. If you know your baby is in pain, hungry, cold, uncomfortable, etc., this takes priority over sleep training and should be addressed.

When to intervene

There may be times when you will want to intervene, like when your baby is crying too hard or too much for your liking, and that is perfectly fine. You can go in and check on your baby using the same approach as you did at bedtime. As long as your baby goes back to sleep on his own, you can check on him as you see fit, keeping in mind the principle of giving your baby enough time to practice independent sleep.

Depending on your baby's age, growth, or stage of development, you may need to feed your baby at night. Please check with your pediatrician on how many feedings your baby should get, if any, and how often you should feed. Knowing this information ahead of time is helpful so you'll know exactly how to handle a waking. If your pediatrician or health advisor believes your baby still needs to eat at night, make sure you keep your baby awake during the feeding, so he is still falling asleep on his own afterwards. This way, you can still teach good sleep habits, even if your baby needs to eat at night.

QUICK FIX Some babies get very sleepy during their night feeding and inevitably fall asleep. If your baby is warm, bundled, and getting his favorite thing in the world, a feeding in your arms, this is a total recipe for sleepy time. Some tricks you can try to keep your baby up include tickling his feet, burping him, uncovering or unzipping his sleep outfit, and lastly, if all else fails, you can change his diaper after the feeding.

If at any point during the sleep training you believe your baby is hungry, sick, or uncomfortable, the sleep training rules go out the window—tend to your baby. Your baby may have visible symptoms like coughing, congestion, vomiting, or fever, or he may have none at all but your parenting gut tells you that something isn't right. Those are all valid reasons to pause the sleep training and give your doc a call to schedule a checkup before resuming.

As your child learns how to sleep by himself, waking up in the middle of the night tends to become less frequent because he will have grown accustomed to not having you or your spouse around when he wakes up in the middle of the night. While your child's still getting to that point, it's highly possible that he will still wake up at night, especially when he still needs you around in order to fall asleep.

During those times, it may be easier to just let your toddler climb on your bed to sleep with you as he still hasn't learned to fall asleep on his own without having to be held. Otherwise, it may just lead to frequently waking up at night. As he starts becoming accustomed to falling asleep just being with you and not touching you, he'll eventually be able to go back to sleep on his own at night without need to wake you up.

If at that point your child does wake you up and needs you at night, then you can start discouraging such behavior by taking your child back to his bed and sitting beside him while he falls back to sleep.

If you're a mom and you're nursing your toddler, it's alright to nurse him at night for as long as you're okay with it. But, as with many other toddlers, it's possible for your child to wake up all night just to ask for milk. In a case such as this, I advise that you start night-weaning your toddler already, which shouldn't adversely affect your nursing relationship. Just ensure that during your child's waking hours, there are lots of nursing opportunities to make up for the lack of milk in the evenings.

One of the best ways to break off the nursing habit at night if you're a mom, is to ask for help from your husband or partner by sending him to your child at night when he wakes up. And if you're strong enough to enforce this strictly, by informing your toddler during the day that you can't come to the rescue at night because you need to rest and that only your husband or partner can do that, your child will slowly learn to accept that and comply. The key here is someone is there to give your child comfort in the night time waking moments.

Reasons Why Your Baby Is Waking Up at Night and Won't Sleep

A baby who is waking up at night is one of the most widely recognized issues parents struggle to enable their baby to survive. One step to understanding how it allows a baby to sleep better at night is to have a superior understanding of why a baby wakes at night. In this chapter, we will feature the five primary reasons for a baby waking up at night.

1. Your baby has a sleep association

Sleep association is otherwise called crutches or sleep props. These include your baby has a specific thing or way that they have been adapted to accept they "need" to have the option to fall asleep. For some babies, this will be a bottle feeding, or breastfeeding, pacifier to sleep. For different babies, this might be some development, for example, rocking, skipping, strolling, or a ride in the vehicle. Some higher needs babies will come to depend on a mix of sleep crutches, for example, jumping with a pacifier.

The age of the baby and the type of sleep association are the two things to think about when deciding the best game-plan to take to help instruct a baby to fall asleep alone and to break his reliance on his sleep crutch. It is additionally a good idea to remember the baby's personality when making a sleep preparing plan.

2. Your Baby is Teething

It may feel like your baby is always teething for a long time, particularly when numerous babies experience teething inconveniences sometimes before a tooth even comes through. When teething appears to make your baby wake more night, it tends to be difficult to tell how to deal with proceeding to show your baby to sleep well. Parents may ponder, "Is my baby in pain?" "Is this why my baby is waking throughout the night?" Often a baby-waking because of teething is a brief stage where a baby will return to their regular sleep habits once they feel better as long as the parents have attempted to remain consistent with putting a baby to sleep as they did before teething and during the teething process. Attempt to have a sleep plan set up for your baby during those teething stages.

3. Baby is eager

Numerous parents are informed that their baby ought not to require feeding during the night after a particular age. This may be valid if each baby were the same and had precisely the same needs. This is mostly not the case. On average, numerous babies will, in any case, need a feeding or two at a half year of age. It is important to remember that 11-13 hours is quite a while for a baby with a little belly to abandon eating. A baby waking at night out of craving can, in any case, be encouraged without making a feeding sleep association and regularly a feed at night is exactly what a baby needs to keep on sleeping through the remainder of the night.

4. Babies are human as well.

While the facts demonstrate that most babies will flourish with a decent timetable and schedule, parents can sometimes lose the point of view and become befuddled that their baby does not sleep the same consistently. Babies are individuals as well, and not robots. They will have some flightiness about them, their characters, and needs. There are a few babies who do sleep and wake predictably however there is similarly the same number of who don't. Like a parent may not be hungry at the very same time each day, a baby may not sleep at the same time every night. Babies will have great days for sleep and awful days like every other person.

There are numerous reasons why a baby can wake at night and with small child sleep issues, at that point number of goals will in general increment. Attempt to understand why your baby might wake at night and after that work to discover an answer, whether it is brief comfort during a troublesome stage or weaning her from a sleep association. As babies develop, they will change and their ability to learn and understand grows significantly. The same will apply to their sleep habits, so it is ideal to attempt to be adaptable and understanding yet consistent when showing your baby how to sleep better.

Manage the Baby Healthy Sleeping Habits

Teaching your child how to sleep alone can be a daunting task, particularly for the parents already exhausted and overwhelmed. For many parents, the cycle of helping a child learn self-catering skills, and finally falling asleep can be emotionally stressful as they take a firm stance in response to the child's protests. The great news is that a child learns this ability very quickly, regardless of age (usually in less than five days). When you have mastered the talent, it's like riding a bike-it's always there. So long as you keep your child sleeping alone, harmful sleep habits will not form as long as you live alone.

Yet healthy sleep habits are controlled, not a one-time fix. This is particularly true for the first five to six years when a child transitions from the basinet to the kid's bed. Three specific areas typically disturb a child's

173

sleepover these years requiring parental management: meeting developmental milestones, getting a snack, and switching from bedside to a bed.

Developmental milestones

Many babies develop sleep problems between the ages of six and nine months. This even extends to those babies who have slept well to this level. Such difficulties are thought to emerge as a result of the cognitive and physical changes currently occurring. Children become more socially aware and understand how their bodies can be manipulated. A kid also begins to turn off his belly a while before he learns to roll back. Many kids will sleep and love lying in their tummy while others wake up and cry out in frustration. Another typical example is a child who knows how to sit down but still doesn't know how to relax. When a parent puts this child into bed, she pulls up to a stand and cries out for help. Of course, if parents keep rolling over their babies or helping their kids sit, it can be an excellent game for the kid quickly!

Parents will deal with these problems in various ways, but a strategy must be determined before the night starts. Keeping to the schedule all night long is just as important. Many parents choose to continue helping their kid until the kid learns the skills needed (e.g., from a stand to a sitting position). Typically the child will take care of himself again within a month. Nonetheless, other parents may feel too exhausting. The faster solution is to let the child figure it autonomously at night. For example, when a child rolls on his belly, the child learns to roll back or sleep on his stomach. The same applies to a kid who makes a stand. The child must finally let go, fall down, and go to sleep. In a crib, this is perfectly safe. Most parents would test their child in intervals without helping the child physically out of his "pickle."

It is essential for parents to understand the age of sleep.

A young baby takes four naps or more a day. She will slowly drop her naps for her first two years before she just takes one. It is half the fight to know when your child is at the age to drop a nap. Once your child reaches this stage, there may be an awkward time when the absence of the fallen rest is too tired. This time should be less than two weeks if timed correctly.

Bed to big kid

Bed For many parents, switching from a crib to a bed is painless, while other people fight with night-time challenges as soon as their child has left a crib. Timing is essential, and it is necessary to have a clear plan. It is not recommended that a child be put to bed before the age of two, except where safety concerns are absolutely necessary. The child will preferably be verbally competent and capable of following the "laws" of moving into a room.

Certain conditions can also influence the sleep habits of an infant. These include holidays or travel, protests, disease, and social activities. If any of these disturbances arise, the sleep cycle should be covered as much as possible. Try to fit most naps on holiday or put your child in bed early in the night. Avoid naps and go to bed late is usually a recipe for an emotionally exhausting holiday. It is essential to get your child back on schedule as soon as possible. The day your child no longer is ill, or the day you return from your trip home, respond to your original sleep and hopes immediately. Your child will protest, but it will be short-lived if you stand firm and consistent.

When your daughter has learned the ability to sleep alone, it is up to you to continually sustain the sleep and ensure that she is well-healed. To ensure continued progress, it is necessary to change the routine in the correct manner of age and not as you need to sleep (like, "I don't want to nap!") or to try to determine sleep as best the family can. It is necessary to return to the normal sleep cycle when disrupted immediately. If you do these things, the bedtime fights will be reduced. The child should know exactly what it wants, which gives her a sense of safety and security.

The management of healthy sleep is a multi-purpose operation. First, parents have to take into account different developmental milestones in young children and develop a plan that helps manage them effectively in terms of sleep. Secondly, parents need to create a dialogue and help the child to self-regulate their sleep need.

If sleep cycles are disturbed because of the holiday, sickness, doctor's appointments, and playing dates, parents need a management plan.

Holiday or Hosting Company

It is a good idea to prepare and schedule how to handle your child's sleep while going out of town. Pack important sleep things that your child likes to have while he is sleeping with him. If your child shares a room with you while traveling, consider how to isolate you from your son. Many rooms have extensive wardrobes, toilets, or small crib-fitting coves. When necessary, find hotel rooms, making it easier to split. Consider bringing a travel noise machine so that your movement and sounds won't interfere with your child while he is sleeping. The other choice is to sleep together for some or all of the night if this allows everyone to sleep better.

Try to honor the sleep schedule of your child as much as possible while traveling. Afternoons can be an excellent time to have a siesta and a quiet time for the whole family. If a nap is missed, try getting your child to bed earlier that night. Keep the patterns for sleep the same as you do at home. This will make your child's transition to sleep much more accessible.

The first whole day or night, you return to your regular routine directly after your journey. At ordinary times, the child should sleep in his crib or bed. He discovers the difference between "holiday sleep" and "home sleep."

When you host the business at home, try to adhere as much as possible to your child's timetable. Also, the more quality your child's sleep gets, the more enjoyable it will be to play and go out.

Illness

If your child is sick, it revolves around its needs. Disease Enables her to sleep when she can and console her in any helpful way. If you want to take your child with you to bed or sleep with her in her room, it's okay. Families must do what works best for the family to sleep as much as possible through the illness. When your child is usually eating and playing, return to your regular sleep schedule immediately. At first, she might argue, but if you're clear and robust, it'll be rapid. Early in the morning, your daughter should understand what happens when she is sick and what is expected of her when she is well.

Miscellaneous Diseases

Try to plan your doctor's appointments, orders, and playdates as far as possible for your child's sleep schedule. Hold five days/week to prepare. It is crucial that parents balance the feeling that their children are stuck in the routine and the sleep needs of their children. If your child takes a morning nap, put it down for the afternoon-nap 15 to 30 minutes earlier. When you miss the afternoon nap, then put your child in bed more prior. In general, as in holidays, it is better not to ignore the child's sleep plan for a whole day, i.e., to skip the naps and to put them to bed very late. It quickly makes it difficult for your child to rebound from this kind of sleep loss and feel very overwhelmed.

When dealing with any sleep disorder, whether it is for a day or for a while, it is essential to return to a regular schedule when you are able to do so. If you do not respond immediately to the plan, the child is confused. Beginning at an early age, babies learn the difference from childhood, healthy sleep from daytime to nighttime sleep, holiday sleep, and illness sleep. If these lines are clearly drawn for every interruption, your child will quickly learn what is anticipated and complain less.

Why Baby Wakes at Night and Won't Sleep

One of the most common problems that parents have to help their baby get rid of is a baby that wakes at night. One move in learning how to help a baby sleep during the night better is to understand why a baby wakes during the night.

Principal explanations for a night waking infant.

I. Your baby has a "Sleep Group" that is also known as "sleep aids" or "crutches," meaning that your baby has a specific product or technique that is conditioned to believe it "needs" to fall asleep. It would be a pacifier, bottle feeder, or breastfeeding for many babies to sleep. This might be any motion like jumping, skipping, walking, or driving in the car for other children. Some babies with higher needs are relying on a combination of sleep crutches as a rebound with a pacifier.

The baby's age and the form of sleeping relationships are both factors to be taken into account when deciding which way to help baby sleep and break its dependence on his sleep crutch. It is also a good idea to take into account the personality of the baby when developing a sleep workout.

II. New developmental milestones All these are developmental milestones that can interrupt your child's sleep at midday, during naptime, when your baby learns how to crawl, pull up, walk, or talk. The main thing that you have to know about sleep disorders related to developmental milestones is to keep you rational because even if your baby doesn't seem to have a new skill, it doesn't mean she doesn't always understand. Also if a developmental milestone can momentarily interfere with your sleep improvement, it does not mean that you still do not know your sleep habits if your sleep training is consistent. Once the baby is old enough to learn how to go back to sleep alone, the waking time at night will be less frequent and less disruptive in the whole family.

III. Your baby is teething. It may feel like your baby is teething for two years continuously, particularly when many children have teething problems long before a tooth even appears. If something seems to make your baby wake more night, it can be challenging to know how to keep your baby asleep. Parents, the wonder, "Is my child painful?" "Is this why my baby wakes all nights?" A baby waking from the teething often becomes a temporary stage in which a baby goes back to their regular sleep habits as long as the parents try to sleep the same way as before and through their teeth. Try to put your baby in a sleep schedule during these teething periods.

IV. Many parents are told that their baby should not need to be fed after a certain age during the night. This could be so if every baby had precisely the same needs. That's just not the case. Most babies still need to be fed an average of two at the age of six months. It is essential to bear in mind that a baby with a small tummy has to go 10-14 hours without food. A baby who wakes out of hunger at night can still be fed without a feeding sleep party, and often, a feed is just what a baby has to sleep throughout the night.

 V. Babies are also individuals.

Although it is true that most babies thrive on good times and routines, occasionally, parents lose focus and get upset that their baby doesn't sleep the same day after the day. Babies are also humans, not machines. You will be unsure about yourselves, your attitudes, desires, and needs. Some babies are sleeping and waking like clockwork, but as many are not. In the same way that a mother may not be hungry every day, a child may not sleep all night at the same time. Babies like everybody else will have good sleep days and bad days.

There are many explanations for why a child will wake at night and sleep issues for babies, so there are many reasons to wake up. Try to understand why your baby could wake in the night and then work to find out whether it is a temporary relief or weaning it from the sleep community during a disruptive process. As babies grow, they change, and their ability to learn and understand significantly increases. The same applies to your sleep habits so that you can continue to be versatile and accommodating, but consistent in teaching your baby how best to sleep.

Chapter 7

Importance Of Feeding

This may sound obvious but getting the correct amount of calories into a baby can sometimes be more difficult than it seems. When you are developing a daytime schedule, it not only the time you put your baby down in his cot that you will need to consider. The amount of calories he is consuming and how often is key.

A three month baby is able to hold much more in his stomach now that he has grown a bit, than when he was a tiny new born fresh into the world. This is excellent news for you, for he can go for longer between feeds.

If you are establishing a routine at the age of three months, the average baby will need 4 to 6 ounces of milk each time he feeds and a total of 32 ounces every 24 hours. This is the same for both breast milk and formula.

The following schedules work well for many parents:

Newborn :2 to 3 ouncesEvery 3 or 4 hours

One month :4 ouncesEvery 4 hours

Two months :4 ounces6/7 feeds in a 24hr period

Four months :4 to 6 ounces6 feeds in a 24hr period

This is a much easier routine to follow with formula-fed babies, for you can control exactly how much your baby is drinking, but with breast-fed babies you may start to notice that your baby will have feeds more frequently during the day, storing up the calories to be able to sleep for longer at night. This follows the same principle, it just may appear in a slightly different schedule to that above.

If your baby is not dropping night feeds, do not worry. All babies are different and develop at different rates. Once they are a little bigger, you can start to try and coax them to feed more during the day so that they will drop feeds at night, but don't force them. It usually takes a breast-fed baby longer to sleep through the night than a formula-fed baby, for they may not be getting the same amount of calories at each feed.

Once your baby is old enough to be weaned, you can begin to introduce some solid foods to bump up their calories. The advice is to wait until they are about six months of age but it can vary from child to child. As long as your baby can sit up with support, has good head control and has lost the tongue-thrust reflex, he can start to experiment with some solid foods.

The tongue-thrust reflex occurs during the first four months of a baby's life, to prevent him from choking. It really is nature's clever little way of making sure he pushes that foreign object out of his mouth, instead of accidentally swallowing it. So be sure to wait until this reflex has gone, before trying to spoon that lovely mushy vegetable medley into your baby's mouth, otherwise it will all end up on the floor or all over your baby's clothes!

For some reason I've noticed that people struggle most when it comes to eating healthy. I suppose we could attribute it to the abundance of genetically engineered, fast, and processed food in grocery stores. The best way to overcome this is to simply throw out all the food that you know is harmful in your house and replace it with foods made of love. The first step is become aware as to what is optimal for the human body. However, at the end of the day something is only going to harm you if you think it is, but when you make a conscious decision to eat healthy organic food it will be abundantly inexpensive for everyone. This will in turn make the world a better place for all of us.

If you want to see fast weight loss results and better health then try switching to a ketogenic diet or in other words an intermittent fasting regime. People who partake in this discipline have amazing results. The method to this diet is to eat within a specific time frame, generally around eight hours out of the day or less. It retrains your body to use fat as an energy source rather than carbs. Another way to improve your health is to stop eating before six or seven p.m. every night to allow optimal digestion and nutrient assimilation.

Science is quickly proving that a plant-based diet is more optimal for the human body. I choose to eat an all raw vegan diet because I've done the research and it can be the healthiest lifestyle if done properly. I find it most optimal for my body. If you desire radiant health then I recommend learning everything you need to know about it before transitioning to this diet. I've read that if humans all became herbivores there would be enough food to feed the entire planet sevenfold, curing starvation. In order for your body to break down food to convert it into energy it must produce digestive enzymes. It takes eighty percent of the bodies energy do this, and the studies show that your body can only produce so many digestive enzymes within one lifespan. Raw plant foods contain digestive enzymes. The fresher they are the more enzymes they contain. If you want quick long lasting energy that will give you energy all day, without the crash, then reach for the fruit and/or raw foods. If you want to lose weight, no matter how much you eat, and have more energy than you've ever had then try transitioning to a raw plant-based diet. It is also very possible to gain weight on a raw vegan diet if you increase your fat and protein intake with intense training and/or weight lifting. They have done studies on the longest-lived people and what they like to eat. The top five longevity foods as a collective include all vegetarian sources as followed: chocolate, cinnamon, red onions, olive oil, and honey. Whatever you eat, opt for organic or homegrown and preferably raw.

Organic foods are important for a number of reasons. They cannot be irradiated or produced with toxic chemicals such as pesticides, herbicides, fungicides, or larvicides. They also cannot be grown from genetically modified seeds. Irradiation is a food preservation process that destroys all the healthy bacteria which is important for the human body; it also has been proven to destroy vital nutrients. Local and homegrown organic fresh fruits and vegetables are the safest as well as most nutritious food options. I eat an avocado a day to help curve nutrient deficiencies because it is such a complete food source. If you've never had one, or don't like them try one

185

with cold pressed olive oil and sea or pink Himalayan salt. It is my favorite food combination. Herbs are so beneficial for the human body. Taking herbs on a daily basis ensure optimum health and help to curb viruses, fungus, and bacteria that are trying to take over the human body.

Chapter 8

Schedule Feeding Timings

When your baby begins sleeping for longer stretches (four or five hours) at night, you'll presumably see that he's ready to drink less regularly, possible changing his eating schedule. What now? A bottle or nursing session like clockwork, for a sum of eight or so feedings for every 24 hours. When he hits this stage, you can attempt to shift his regular schedule to times that work best for you, creator of From First Kicks to First Steps and Feeding Baby Green. If your tyke drinks from you for a considerable amount of time or nips from a bottle throughout the day, talk to your pediatrician about gradually expanding the time between feedings so your baby will drink more at each meal. Consider giving your little child a pacifier between feeds, as well; some children need to suck a great deal.

Many moms, however, appreciate the round-the-clock closeness that demand feeding involve and accept that their infants profit from their immediate responsiveness. If that is you, there's no need to change what you're doing. If you're formula-feeding, be mindful so as not to overfeed (it's simpler for breastfed infants to self-direct their intake); Dr. Greene's standard guideline is to offer your baby a few ounces of formula for each pound of his body weight, up to a maximum of 32 ounces daily. If your baby is crying from appetite, obviously you wouldn't deprive him. In any case, if a schedule makes for a calmer, more joyful, more rested baby, go for it. Your baby needs you taking care of business.

But somewhere in the range of 4 and six months, your child's sensory system disentangles from its tangled infant mass and composes itself...and he may be ready to soothe himself to sleep. The problem is, your little person presently will not go down except if he's had a seemingly endless amount of your pre-sleep, calming consideration. And that is when many exhausted guardians decide to sleep train. Sleep preparing has many different forms. Be that as it may, the fundamental idea is this: Put your baby down tired, yet alert. If he cries, whisper and rub his back to support him. Leave for a couple of minutes and then come back to soothe him if he's still upset. Repeat until he nods off. Every night, extend the time you let him cry by a couple of minutes until it doesn't happen anymore. Although nobody likes to hear their baby cry, advocates accept that a couple of last nights are justified, despite all the trouble if your child can get more uninterrupted rest time.

Chapter 9

Take Care Of Mom

You may think that the focus of this book is the toddler, but you'd be wrong. I have seen many marriages become less successful because all of the attention is given toward the toddler and the parents have actually put themselves out of the picture. The parent's needs are as important because a tired parent will not be a very patient one. The strength of the relationship also makes the family for the toddler a lot more secure so if both parties are happy, then the toddler will be happier too. However, how do you balance out parent responsibilities with actually allowing yourself the person freedom that you both need?

The home - You do need to strike a happy balance here and if you and your partner can get together to work out duties that can be done on an everyday basis, this really helps. There will be cleaning to be done and the neater you can keep your home, the easier all of these tasks become. If you and your partner can learn to put things away after you have finished with them, this helps to make the home safer for the toddler too. It's good fun to do things like this together. Invest in a dishwasher as it's a major argument that should be doing the dishes. This makes it easier to get menial tasks out of the way. You also need to invest in a good laundry room with plenty of hanging space, so that laundry becomes easier. The child's clothing will cause you a lot of extra washing and you and your partner can take it in turns to wash and hang out the clothes, both taking responsibility for things that are not that much fun to do.

The other thing that you need to decide is how to split money and spare time. I know you will think it a joke when I mention spare time, but with many people telecommuting, working from home is a real possibility, which puts more money in your pockets to actually enjoy yourselves more. Having a child is not the end of the social life as you knew it and you need to be able to relinquish responsibility sometimes and make sure that you have plenty of "us" time. Go on a weekly date or visit friends without the toddler in tow because it's important that the main caregiver of the child has time with adults. It can become very dull indeed when the only person there is to talk to is a toddler!

As your children get older, you need to strike some kind of deal with your partner that you are both on the same page as far as any kind of parenthood goes. If a toddler gets the impression that he can get something out of dad that he can't get out of mom, believe me, he will use this leverage to make his life more fun, but it's likely to drive a wedge between you and your partner. You need to be always on the same page so that there is no doubt in the toddler's mind that he has the upper hand.

The worry of leaving toddler with others

This can become a huge weight on your shoulders if you allow it to become one. The best way to arrange for a babysitter or for your parents to get involved with the toddler is to have a very established routine and to make sure that all people who will care for the child adhere to it. Explain the necessity of regular bedtimes. Talk about what is acceptable and what is not acceptable, because the problem here is that when people step into a new routine, it can be very hard for parents to get the child back to the original routine when the child comes home. Write out a schedule and unless you are certain that those looking after the child will stick to it, find alternatives.

One of the biggest bugbears to the relationship is the fact that baby gets all of the attention. Therefore, it's important for couples to spend enough time with one another and to carry on the relationship even though baby is also part of it now. Sharing the growing up pains and joys is something that's very special indeed and you can keep in touch these days by text or even by Skype when you are absent from one another. Remember, just because you are stuck at home with a toddler doesn't mean that you cannot claim time for yourself. If you want exercise classes, why not time them in with the afternoon nap? If you want to continue to work from home, as long as you can separate things in your life in a reasonable way, there's no reason why you cannot achieve this. You just need to remember that the child does come first because the child needs guidance. However, if you organize your home in such a way that you are able to look over your child while you work, then you may be able to find a good balance and be able to continue working and contributing financially to the relationship. This takes a little pressure off your partner and means that he will be able to spend more time at home with you enjoying watching your child grow up.

You need social interaction. You also need to feel that you have friends so don't make the mistake of giving up contact with friends just because you have a toddler. Okay, those friends may not be into toddler talk, but you can trade evenings with your partner, so that you each get time with your friends as well as being homebound parents. That way, you retain the balance and are a happier and more balanced parent for your child. A parent who begrudges giving up her life to motherhood often carries a lot of bitterness with her and you may not think so now, but kids can pick up on this. It also doesn't help the dynamics of the relationship if you harbor resentment, rather than adjusting your lives to suit both you and your child.

Of all of the toddlers that I looked after during times of crisis, I remember those that came from couples who were actually happy together as being the easiest children to put to bed at night. That's because in their little minds, they harbored no doubts about who mommy and daddy were or the role that they played in their lives. Even though these were foster kids, I can tell you that their lives were defined by who they knew their parents to be and if the parents loved each other and loved their child, the child managed to sleep much better than those poor kids whose parents were unhappy and in the process of separation. The happier you are, the happier your kid will be, so celebrate life and let your toddler see you as a happy and fulfilled human being he/she can respect and love as well as rely upon for positive feedback and learning.

Chapter 10

Take Care Of Proper Nutrition

You can raise an adventurous eater capable of having a healthy and positive relationship with food. Many parents focus on nutrition alone. They focus on the numbers of nutrition—eating 5 fruits and vegetables each day, drinking X amount of breast milk or formula ounces per day, or eating the recommended daily calories. Parents should pay attention to nutrition. After all, it is vital for growth and development. The problem occurs when parents focus too much on the numbers. Nutrition is just one component of healthy eating. Parents should also concentrate on variety of foods and lifelong healthy eating behaviors.

•Teach "flavor preference" by exposing children to a variety of food, texture, and taste through a sensory-rich diet.

•Teach infants and children to recognize and appropriately respond to their feelings of hunger and fullness.

•Maximize nutrient absorption and intake by offering children a variety of nourishing foods.

Teaching Flavor Preference

Flavor preference is taught by offering infants and children sensory-rich foods to eat and explore (you'll read more about this later) starting in infancy.

Most of us only think about our taste buds when we eat something with an intense flavor such as sweet, sour, bitter, or salty. We might also think about taste when we eat something we like or dislike. How often do you consider your baby's taste buds, or even your own? As parents we may overlook the sense of taste because we are so busy trying to be the best parents possible. We are occupied with teaching numbers, letters, words, animals, colors, and songs. Unfortunately, when we feed our children, we tend to concentrate on how much the child is eating, more than the elements that make up the world of flavor.

Parents are faced with many personal decisions without realizing the long-term impact they can have on a child's eating behavior. Tiny taste buds begin to form in the fetus, and further develop in infancy. The food choices we make while pregnant, breastfeeding, and during meals have the potential to expose an infant to a variety of foods. A pregnant or lactating mother's food choices mold a child's food preferences. Breast milk emits the aroma and flavors of the mother's diet. If a pregnant or breast feeding mother eats garlic, the child will taste garlic. If she eats curry, the child will taste curry. If she eats cumin, the child will taste cumin. Even more fascinating is that the infant will remember the taste of those flavors after birth, encouraging food acceptance in later months and years.

One of the first choices you can make that will influence the infant's food preferences is the decision to breastfeed. The American Academy of Pediatrics (AAP), Institute of Medicine, and World Health Organization (WHO) all stress the benefits of exclusive breastfeeding for the first 6 months. Breastfed infants are more likely to accept new foods during the first introduction compared to a formula fed infant. This is understandable because a formula fed infant experiences one bland flavor day in and day out.

Breastfeeding is instrumental to the introduction of a variety of tastes. The longer a child is breastfed, the more apt the child is to eat fruits and vegetables later in life. Therefore, lactating women are encouraged to eat a varied diet.

As the child transitions to solid foods, the mother can continue to teach flavor preference by offering a variety of food. The more variety of food offered to the infant at 6 months of age, the better the acceptance of new foods. The overall feeding experience of the fetus, infant, and child is heavily influenced by the dietary patterns and decisions of the caregivers.

Let's back up a minute and define the term variety. Most parents tend to associate variety with the idea of introducing different foods (asparagus, banana, apple, carrot). However, there is more to variety. If a child does not like carrots one day, don't give up. Just cut or prepare them differently the next time you serve carrots. In other words, carrots can be cut into long spears, coined, mashed, or diced. The idea of providing variety is not limited to serving new foods, but offering the same foods different ways.

As the child becomes accustomed to the food he will be more apt to try it. Children will eat what is familiar to them. It is the parent's job to make the food familiar to the child through multiple introductions. However, it is important to ensure the texture of the food is age- and skill-appropriate .

A Sensory-Rich Diet

The basis of "flavor preference" is exposing the child to a variety of food by providing a sensory feeding experience. Sensory-rich food offers a variety of tastes, mouthfeel, and aroma while feeding in the appropriate balance. Food provides an opportunity for a child to use all of his senses (taste, touch, smell, sound, and sight). The acceptance or refusal of the meal is determined by those senses. Not only does the flavor of the food bring either disappointment or enjoyment, but the environment also determines the acceptance of the food. Depending on the child, a slight or drastic change in one aspect of the meal can change the entire experience. An uncomfortable seat, a very hot room, or an over-spiced dish can negatively impact the child's experience. It is important to consider all of the senses when creating a positive feeding experience.

Every adult knows the type of foods they like and do not like. Children are no different. They too have opinions about food, and also have stronger and more sensitive taste buds than adults, because unfortunately, adults lose taste buds as they age. Keep in mind—what an adult tastes is completely different than what a child tastes.

Parents should expose children to a variety of foods, but they should also respect their children's individual sensory preferences. Some children will be very sensitive to taste or texture (maybe even both). For example, my son had and still has a texture issue. He hated lumps in his yogurt. I learned to respect this preference and avoided lumps in creamy textures. He is now three and I continue to make slow changes in the texture of his food. Parents can determine an individual starting point for their child by simply listening to the child's verbal or nonverbal language. This might take time to see a pattern. If you can recognize a food aversion early and work slowly around it, you will be ahead of the game.

If you have a sensitive child, go slow. Mild, diluted, or smooth food may be more inviting to a sensitive child. Don't worry—all hope is not lost if your child dislikes a lump in their yogurt or cinnamon in their applesauce. It's just a starting point. Again, start slow and make very small changes. Select foods the child enjoys and add **very** small changes to the sensation. Avoid sensory surprises for the sensitive child—it would not be a good idea to give her plain scrambled eggs one day and a southwestern omelet the next. Just changing the amount of milk added to the eggs is enough sensory change to start with.

Remember that all children are different. They are different from adults, other children, and even themselves. Children change constantly. Their flavor preference will also change day to day. Just because a child liked a specific texture or flavor one day, does not mean she will like it the next.

This is common behavior and should be accepted as normal, not picky (we will discuss this later).

Taste

Bitter, salty, sour, sweet, and umami (savory) are the 5 senses our taste buds recognize. Every nourishing bite will provide your baby with one taste or a combination of tastes which all influence each other. For example, something sweet can reduce the bitter taste of a vegetable. Knowing how to provide foods to maximize and balance flavor will encourage children to eat their vegetables. In other words, if you want your infant to benefit from the nutrients in a bitter food like leafy greens, you can add a sweet fruit like a banana to make the flavor more accepting. This is called "flavor pairing."

Let's face it—human babies naturally refuse bitter foods and welcome sweet and salty foods. It is not their fault—it is imbedded deep into their DNA. Our ancestors' survival was dependant upon their ability to distinguish between bitter and sweet foods. The most poisonous foods taste very bitter, making them unappealing. However, the sensation of bitter and sweet can vary considerably between each person due to age and genetics. Parents and children naturally have different taste senses and can influence the perceptions of picky eating as well. The good news is that flavor preference is learned, and strong flavors can be accepted over time.

Not only do infants prefer sweet foods but they are also neophobic (fear of something new) about food. They have an inherent ability to protect themselves from potentially toxic foods. Don't worry—just because they fear new foods and love sweet foods, doesn't mean they can't learn to be healthy eaters. If your baby scowls at the taste of something new, don't give up after a couple introductions. Keep moving forward and concentrate on your willingness to reintroduce the same foods. Just change the flavor. Remember, changing the flavor is a simple as changing the texture (mash, finely dice, chop), adding an herb or spice, or serving it at a different temperature.

Myth Buster: Many pediatricians, grandmothers, and mothers recommend giving infants vegetables before fruit. It is thought that the sweet taste of fruit will interfere with the preference for bitter vegetables. There isn't any clear evidence supporting this theory. In fact, a variety of fruits and vegetables during pregnancy and breastfeeding lead to a greater acceptance of those foods by the infant. Also, repeated exposure to fruits and vegetables during weaning creates a preference.

Mouthfeel

Texture, Shape, and Temperature

Our mouth has the ability to feel. It can distinguish textures and temperatures, which can have a dramatic impact on the flavor of our food. A food's texture has the ability to captivate and satisfy us at the same time. Creamy, fatty foods give us comfort, while crunchy foods give us pleasure at a social event. However, a food's texture can also repulse us. I know several adults who do not like texture combinations of creamy and lumpy.

Keep this in mind when feeding your little one. They have opinions about texture, too.

Infants and children commonly refuse new foods because they may not like the texture or the taste of the food. Parents tend to perceive this behavior as "picky." There are a couple common mistakes parents can make when introducing a new food to their child. Temperature also affects the perception of a food's taste. It makes food more enjoyable, and can bring out the sweetness or even hide the bitterness of food. For example, letting ice cream sit out on the counter for a few minutes before serving will maximize its sweet taste. Even better—freezing bitter vegetables will take the bitter taste out of your smoothie when it is blended frozen and consumed immediately!

Infants should be introduced to a variety of temperatures, including cold, cool, warm, and tepid. Parents should avoid serving foods that are too hot— a baby's mouth is more sensitive than an adult's, and it is important to use caution. If a food feels slightly hot to you, err on the safe side and cool it more for your baby.

Chapter 11

Try To Balance Your Sleep With Newborn

Sleep deprivation is part of being a parent, but it can definitely put a toll on you and your health if it goes on for months. So to help you survive this stage in your life, I have listed some tips that you can follow to help you compensate your sleep.

Eat healthily – It is really challenging to function as an adult, and even more challenging to take care of your little one, if you don't have enough sleep. One way to guarantee that you have enough energy to survive the day is to eat a healthy breakfast.

 Aim to have a plate with protein (such as chicken or eggs), whole grains (oats, brown rice, whole-wheat bread, etc.) and fresh fruit. You may want to avoid high-sugar foods as these will only deplete your energy after a while.

Drink lots of water – Your body needs water so that it can properly function. Make sure that you get enough water (more than 8 glasses) to also avoid getting sick. You don't want to be ill while taking care of your baby.

Sleep when your baby sleeps – This was a piece of advice given to me that I am so thankful for. Avoid the need to watch your baby while s/he sleeps

(I know most new parents know what I mean) and try to get some shut-eye while your little one is dozing off. This could help you get through the long nights of trying to get him/her to sleep.

Ask for help – Consider asking for help from your parents or in-laws, especially when you think you're getting too overwhelmed and exhausted. I'm pretty sure they'll be more than willing to watch over their grandchild during the day while you get your much-needed rest.

Unplug – Some parents may find it tempting to check on their mobile phones or laptops when their baby is asleep to at least get a taste of the "outside" world. If it is not that important, try to unplug and get some sleep yourself. Believe me, you need sleep more than you need to get updates from your social media feed.

Sleep train your child – Start planning on sleep training your child when s/he is ready. Sleep training, when it works, really helps parents to get quality sleep.

Sleeping All Through the Day

When it comes to the baby's need for rest, there is no certain standard. You must be sharp and attentive with regards to the rest needs of your child. There are no exact standards regarding how long the baby should rest. In any case, you will see that in an initial couple of days and long stretches of his life, he will spend most of his time sleeping. There will be times when he will be conscious, even amidst the night, although if your child is like most, these frequencies will be far in the middle. In any case, indeed soon, you will find that he will build up an individual rest pattern. Do the trick it to state that at this phase in his life, rest is his best technique for development. So, you need to alter your resting pattern too if you are to guarantee your baby's development.

The Baby is the Center of Things

During the first days and long stretches of his life, your baby ought to be the focal point of your life. That is why if you are a working mother, it would genuinely be savvy to plan your maternity leave for a month or two until you can securely endow your child to a parental figure. During your leave, you can utilize your time by being centered around your baby's needs. In any case, this doesn't imply that you disregard your own physical needs. What's more, something that you ought not to ignore is having the right amount of rest, regardless of whether you are troubled by the baby's cries very early on.

Understanding Baby Sleep Patterns

Getting used to having a newborn baby can be difficult for parents. The biggest change for most parents can be getting acclimated with baby sleep patterns. It is an indisputable fact that new parents can expect numerous sleepless nights, so understanding what kind of sleep their baby will get might help parents to acknowledge what these initial couple of months will look like.

A newborn baby, generally, does little more than sleep and eat. This keeps mother occupied with breastfeeding and nonstop diaper changes. Baby sleep patterns for the initial three weeks ought to be an aggregate of 16-20 hours of sleep each day. Since they will sleep for around 2 hours at a time, this means parents may almost certainly take short naps for the initial three weeks or should sleep in shifts. At three weeks, the baby will start sleeping 16 to 18 hours a day, maybe sleeping for more extended periods. At six weeks, the baby will sleep even less, around 15 to 16 hours a day. This means parents could expect to sleep a little more at this age.

The age of four months means the baby will sleep 9 to 12 hours at night in addition to 2 naps during the day. Parents will cheer as baby sleep patterns, at last, enable them to get an entire night's sleep. Throughout the following couple of months, the baby will keep on having increasingly stable sleep patterns and offer parents a truly necessary break from interfering with sleep. These baby sleep patterns are fundamental for baby to get the nourishment and solace she needs to grow properly. Trying to understand what's in store at different stages can help set up the unseasoned parents for the sleep they will almost certainly get as a baby develops.

Polyphasic Sleep

Also known as Uberman's Sleep Schedule, this method of sleeping changes your sleeping patterns but doesn't cut out on the necessary quality rest that your body needs.

The usual pattern of sleeping is known as biphasic. That means there are two phases for sleep within a 24-hour block. With that being said, polyphasic sleep pertains to sleeping several times a day.

With polyphasic sleep, you want your body to make that dive but only for about 2 hours.

The core approach of polyphasic sleeping is to break down your full resting period for a day into 4 to 6 sleep periods, each being about 2 hours long. This may sound like a crude approach to cutting corners on sleep, but it's a crude method that works.

How it Works

Take note that the body doesn't necessarily have to experience a full 8 hours of sleep to start recuperating and healing. It just has to be in the right state while you sleep. Normally, that takes time as you go through each cycle.

With polyphasic sleep, you start telling your body that you will no longer be able to get a full 8 hours of sleep. Instead, you're replacing your full 8 hours with smaller 2-hour chunks that happen frequently throughout the day.

Depending on how long your body takes to get the hint, you could be looking at 2 weeks until your body realizes that a full 8 hour block of sleeping is never happening.

When this happens, your body will begin to adjust to your new pattern of sleeping by injecting as much brain activity in your new (and limited) sleep time as possible. This will allow you to wake up refreshed and energized after a mere two hours of sleep.

Benefits

Naturally, this method works great for people who have very little control over the time they get to sleep. Professionals that need to be on-call for emergencies will now have the energy to do what they have to do without sacrificing their good night's sleep.

This sleeping pattern also allows you to do more within the day, especially if you're more inclined to do things when you're supposed to be sleeping. The flexibility that this method provides you allows you more space in which to plot out your daily activities instead of squeezing everything into a single day.

Baby and Mother Sleeping Habits

If you are a new mother, you must understand the right mother and baby sleeping habits to ensure your child's proper growth and development. Nonetheless, your baby's development should not be your primary concern, as you are the principal source of life support to the baby. You should also have the right amount of sleep to fulfill your physical needs correctly.

All-day Sleeping

There is no hard and fast rule when it comes to the baby's need to sleep. You have to be vigilant and careful about your child's sleep needs. There are no stringent rules on how long the baby will sleep. But you will find that he will spend most of his time relaxing in the first few days and weeks of his life. Of course, occasionally, even in the middle of the night, he's waking up, however, if your child is healthy, these incidences are far between. But you will soon find that he is going to develop a regular pattern of sleep. It's enough to assume that sleep is his best method of growth at this stage of his life. You must, therefore, also change your sleep patterns if you are to ensure the success of your infant.

The baby is the core of everything.

The baby should be the subject of your life during the first days and weeks of his life. This is why if you're a working mother, it's really nice to plan a motherhood leave for a month or two until you can comfortably trust a caregiver to your son. You will make the best use of your time during your vacation by centralizing your baby's needs. But you don't neglect your own physical needs. So one thing you should not forget is getting the right amount of sleep, even if in the wee hours of the morning you get distracted by the baby's cry.

Put the right mother and baby sleeping habits.

While children are unique, at this early stage of their life, they have a common need. They all need a lot of time to sleep. This is one of the ways of nature to make safe and active children. And here, you can get your child to sleep well-by leading your child to develop good sleep habits. Therefore, you also have the right amount of rest to give him adequate nutrition (in the form of breast milk) for his healthy development.

You should start deciding what the best time to sleep for you and your baby is. If your routine is early to sleep, you can try to get your baby to sleep approximately one hour earlier. We also know that most children are busy and must be coaxed and soothed prior to sleep. This one-hour system is for that reason only. If you don't, you will find your sleep is late, so you will be robbed of your much-needed rest.

You should also be worried about his daytime sleep. No issue if you're still on vacation because you can spend all of your time with your son. But when you really have to go back to work, there are complications if your child simply takes his own time to sleep. Therefore, sleeping him frequently throughout the day-perhaps one in the morning and one in the afternoon is a good practice. This way, the caregiver has no problem putting your child to sleep when you leave him.

We cannot see it, but there are definitely a lot of things going on during sleep. And in kids, this is very evident. Also, wonder why children who always sleep have round bodies-but have sluggish reactions against external stimuli almost always? This emphasizes that sleep should not be overdone. When you follow your mother and baby's proper sleep patterns, the child's body and mind are both safe, and this goes with you.

Chapter 12

Learn Your Responsibilities

In children, any request of which is immediately fulfilled, the requests increase in increasing order until they cross all reasonable boundaries or even become unacceptable. What is he doing? It is time for the adult to tell him: "Stop it—you are already going too far. No means no."

Your one-year-old baby mumbles something half asleep. Then, for no reason, he begins to scream or cry. You come to check what happened, but at first glance, everything is in order. You think that he is hungry, and a bottle of warm milk will calm him. Indeed, the child falls asleep again. He thinks to himself: "Great, a bottle of milk, but I didn't even ask for anything, just shouted a little, how simple it is! Why not ask for another one tomorrow too? Or even two. It's so nice to drink milk on daddy's hands in the middle of the night."

So the next time you feel a "trap," just say no. But how to make this crybaby who does not want to listen obey, and it seems as if he is really suffering?

Everything is very simple: you want to sleep peacefully at night, your child wants something else (to spend most of the night playing with you, or sleep on your hands). You have convincing logical and biological arguments that he doesn't even want to listen to: "To grow up, you need to sleep at night, and it's already dark outside." His arguments are loud, heartbreaking,

209

annoying, and incredibly effective. This is his only way to formulate his requests. Your child knows what he wants and is trying to make you understand this by crying. If you do not confront him and resort to his room at the first sob, what do you think will happen?

If you do not teach your child to obey or understand that "no" means "no," then you will not be able to get enough sleep at night for a long time.

Flexible "No"

Flexible "no" means "no," which, if the child continues to insist, eventually turns into "yes." Your baby should understand what the words you say mean. Many children do not simply accept "no" as the answer, as they are used to the fact that something else follows.

If you have accustomed your child to the fact that your "no" means either "not now, wait," or "ask again," or "shout louder and see," then do not be surprised that he does not listen.

Better to say:

"Yes. Yes, but this is the last time. No."

Than:

"No. No. Well, good, but only this time—yes."

You thought that you said no, you gave a convincing reason for your refusal. This is quite enough. After you say: "No, I won't bring you a third time in the evening to drink," do not come back. Otherwise, what do you think will happen the next day?

The Tone of the Voice Must Match the Words Spoken

What tone do you use to say no to your child? After all, for the most part, it will be precisely by your intonation that he will evaluate how determined you are in your words. So let him know that you are not joking.

"No," you need to speak in a strict and clear voice, but do not shout. Show by the tone of voice, gestures, and eyes that you are not joking and are not going to change your mind.

Parents who firmly know what they want behave around the child in a very calming and encouraging way, even if at first the refusal causes him temporary resentment.

Control Your Emotions

A small child is very susceptible to everything that happens around him; he sees everything like a video camera. All the accumulated information is deposited in his head. If what he saw seems to him particularly interesting, then he tries to repeat it.

When a child is born, he does not know how to control neither his emotions nor their apparent manifestation. For a long period, he can demonstrate his disagreement only with a cry or shout. If you also shout at him because you can no longer tolerate this, then he will never learn to control his emotions, and nights in your family will turn into hell.

Set an Example

This method of teaching new behavior is called imitation, and animals have been using it for a long time: the one who does not know how to do something watches the one who knows how, and tries to repeat it until he does the same. Such training takes place silently but is extremely effective.

Nobody makes you behave perfectly. It is important to constantly remember that parents are the first role model for their children, the first authority, the people they love and respect the most by their children. Therefore, you exert the greatest influence on the child.

How are you going to teach your child to be quiet at night, if, at the same time, you yourself allow yourself to shout at him? These children should adopt the model of parental behavior and not vice versa. If a fit of anger infuriates you, then everything turns upside down.

If you want the child to stop screaming, then you yourself should not scream at him.

Staying Calm

Parents work a lot; they have a lot of things to do and very little time to complete them. This keeps them tense, with virtually no stopping. And most often, children suffer from this, who themselves are at the limit of fatigue and everything experienced during the day. After all, oftentimes, their whims become that very "last straw.".

It's hard for any person to stay calm all the time. In order to learn to control your anger, it is important to clearly understand that there is no "guilt" of the child in this. He only "sets fire to the fuse."

Everyone is responsible for their emotions and for how they express them. Parents who get angry must cope with their anger. Children, in turn, have to deal with their own!

Violations of children's sleep (for example, when a baby gets out of bed twenty times a night, instead of sleeping soundly) can cause a flash of rage in parents. This could start a big quarrel. Sometimes, parents get so tired that they tear off the stress that they cannot defuse on their child.

Do not forget:

A child can overcome his own outbursts of anger only thanks to the example he takes from you;

You can reassure your child and become an authority for him only if you remain calm, strict, and at the same time, kind.

Yes, it's not so simple. However, do not lose your patience! You can fix it.

Confusing Needs and Whims

"If I don't react to the cries of my child at night, how can I be sure that everything is fine with him?"

Young children have their own needs, and it is very important to satisfy them. Fortunately, there are not so many of them. The problem is that a child with the same zeal expresses not only his needs but also just desires, so parents sometimes confuse these two concepts with each other.

Each child has its own obvious needs, familiar to every parent. First comes the primary needs that must be met in the first place—the need for food and water, warmth, and care. Next comes the social needs—to be approved and looked after. Then comes the need for protection—it is important for the baby to feel that he has not been abandoned or rejected. Next comes the mental needs—to play, study, and discover something new. Finally, the child needs to be surrounded by an environment that allows him to develop correctly and give all his best.

Each child should receive all of the above.

Pleasure Principle

The child believes that his pleasure is the most important thing; therefore, it comes to the point that he requires the immediate implementation of any of his whim. He doesn't just want to get everything that he sees (fire truck, pacifier, pens), he needs it right here and now. It is difficult for him to cope with the emerging sense of injustice when he does not receive just what he wanted or does not receive it right away.

Your task is to refuse the child gradually to fulfill some of his desires, but at the same time not to go too far so that he begins to understand what life is. If this is not done, then life itself will correct it; however, in this case, the child will have a hard time.

If you indulge in any desires of your baby, then you will render him only a disservice.

Here are a few examples to make a difference:

Hug your baby more often. But if a child wants to spend fifteen hours a day on pens, then this is a whim.

The child needs to eat; this is his need. If at six months he wants a bottle of milk before bedtime, then this is a whim.

Sleeping in warmth is a need. Sleeping between dad and mom is a whim.

The child needs to be escorted to bed. This is a need. If he calls his mother ten times a night, this is nothing but a whim.

Failure or Frustration

The child suffers from unsatisfying basic needs, and the consequences of his suffering can seriously affect his future life. We often see problems in adults who, in childhood, lacked care, love, or stability in their relationship with their parents.

The desire should not be immediately satisfied. It should be heard and understood - with tenderness and empathy. If this is followed by a refusal, then its reason must be clearly formulated. Does the child not like this? Does he show his displeasure loudly? Nothing wrong.

Children become screamers and little tyrants just when all their desires and whims are constantly being fulfilled. They continue to search for the limits of what is permitted but still cannot find them.

Getting Rid of Guilt

Feeling guilty is very persistent, and it is very difficult to get rid of it. It often appears in parents trying to cope with sleep disturbances in a child. It can take various forms: parents feel guilty for leaving their baby to cry alone, for allowing him to come to the parental bed, as they can't teach him how to sleep normally.

Feelings of guilt arise from the feeling that we did something wrong, but this is not always true. It's in vain to say to yourself "I should have" or "I should have done" - you won't help the matter with self-flagellation. The most effective way to get rid of guilty feelings, as practice shows, is to switch to active actions.

If you are making any attempt to improve the child's sleep, then there is no need to doubt yourself: the more you are confident in your actions, the less space will be left for guilt.

If thoughts of guilt visit you, then you should understand the following:

If a child cries instead of sleeping or constantly wakes up in the middle of the night, then everything is not okay with him. Your task, in this case, is to accustom him to a normal sleep mode.

When children get enough sleep, they become calmer, more energetic; they are more open to learning.

Your child does not need you to be around the clock; he just needs to know that you are nearby and love him.

Your child has the right to express anger or protest at some point; you do not need to blame yourself for this.

The best gift you can give your child is to teach him to calm down and sleep alone. This is a great start to develop its independence further.

To put an end to quarrels in the evenings, to become parents who greet the morning with a smile and completely rested - isn't this the most important thing for your child? And do not forget: you also have the right to a night's rest.

People who are naturally very kind are especially vulnerable to guilt. They do not want to disturb others or make them feel bad, and even more so, it concerns their own child. If this is about you, then ask yourself the following question: would you interfere with your child if he tried to cut off his finger with a knife? In the same way, we can say:

If we do not teach the child to sleep normally, then we will allow him to make a mistake.

Finally, do not forget that guilt can develop into anger and aggression, as it leads to internal conflict: we want the child to sleep better at night, but at the same time, we are not ready to do anything for this or to do business with consequences. As a result, one of the two - your spouse or the child himself - will become a victim of such feelings. This will neither help improve the general atmosphere in the house nor solve the problems with your baby's sleep.

Help Each Other

It is very important that both parents take an equal part in solving problems with the baby's sleep. If you do it together, then everything happens calmer, you have more patience, you are more convincing, and you have more strength.

Lack of sleep depletes the nervous system. Not surprisingly, having a baby is a huge test for any couple. It often happens that difficulties with laying a child result in serious marital disagreements. The child understands all this perfectly and feels his responsibility and guilt, and he does not need to bear this heavy burden.

It also often happens that parents, who usually get along very well, start to quarrel when it comes to sleep problems in their child. One of them takes a stricter position: for example, he believes that the child should be left to cry, no longer wants to calm him down, and wants to enjoy a quiet evening or a night's sleep. The other behaves "kinder" with the child, worries that something is wrong with him, that the baby feels abandoned.

Additionally, if a crack forms between the parents, then the child immediately "slips" into it. He quickly becomes a subject of quarrels: as a rule, a stricter parent believes that the second nullifies all his efforts to educate. However, neither authoritarianism nor permissiveness will bring the desired result.

So what to do?

Try not to argue about this in front of the child if the situation is heating up. In any case, do not show him that you do not agree with each other.

Do not let the child get the impression that he can receive from his mother everything that his father just refused (or vice versa). It is because of this that we run the risk of hearing from the bed: "No, dad, call mom!" This parenting error is very difficult to eliminate in the future.

When one of the parents makes a decision, it is advisable that the second does support him in this, even if he does not completely agree with him. If the dispute cannot be avoided, then postpone the clarification of the relationship at a more convenient moment.

When you need to teach your child something new, it is important that both parents are in solidarity with each other: "Mom said no, then no."

Pass the Baton

If parents do not have enough night sleep, it is important that they monitor the child in turn. Pass the baton of the night watch to each other, but continue to act together. Keeping each other in the know, you can ensure that the child is used to the model of behavior you have chosen and the requirements that apply to him.

If you act on one side together or in turn and stick to your plan for a sufficiently long time, then, in the end, the child will learn to behave as you expected.

Chapter 13

Periodic Limb Movement Disorder And Its Treatments

Another sleep disorder which makes the limbs move during sleep is PLMD or periodic limb movement disorder. This happens at different times during the night when the hand and leg extremities experience rhythmic movements.

If you are suffering from PLMD and you wish to treat it, then you need to visit your doctor and have him officially diagnose that you are experiencing this sleep disorder. He will then prescribe different treatment options for the symptoms of PLMD.

Your doctor may advise you to avoid substances that will aggravate PLMD. These may include alcohol and caffeine as they make the limbs move severely while you sleep.

Your physician may prescribe anticonvulsant medications to treat PLMD. There is a possibility that he will prescribe medications intended for Parkinson's disease as these will significantly decrease the gravity of your PLMD symptoms.

Ask your doctor if you can use sleeping aids should you not want to take anticonvulsant medications. Some doctors who may prescribe medications to insure you have a deeper sleep.

After you have taken prescription medicines, visit your doctor again for follow up. He may adjust the dosage previously given to you or he may alter your medications depending on your present state.

When Do Sleep Disorders Begin?

First, I want to take time to make sure you understand that sleeping disorders are not often the fault of either parent. Sleep disorders happen for a variety of reasons and often because the child has an overactive imagination or simply can't adjust to a change of scenery. Babies often suffer through separation anxiety, which can cause a sleep problem and develop into a sleep disorder. Because these factors of life simply happen to your child, as they do with anyone's child, it is extremely important never to take any of these sleeping disorders personally. The more you let your child's sleeping disorder affect you, the harder it will be for your child to overcome the disorder. As parents, our guilt is often high. While I can't tell you not to feel any guilt, I can tell you to find your own techniques to help you work through any guilt or doubts so you can help your child overcome their sleeping disorder.

Many parents don't think their baby is old enough to develop a sleeping disorder. Unfortunately, this thinking is wrong. Your child can develop a sleep disorder as early as a few months old. In fact, sleep disorders in young children are growing. According to a recent study, as many as two out of every three children aged ten and younger have a sleeping disorder. Because of this recent development, doctors have started to discuss the importance of setting up naptime and bedtime routines as this has proven to help your child fight off any sleep disorders. It is important to note that sleep disorders don't always start because the child doesn't get a good night's sleep. While this can be a factor, such as getting used to staying up later or being able to fall asleep when and where they feel like it, there are a lot of other causes of sleep disorders, such as psychological or emotional reasons.

On top of studying the causes of sleep disorders in children, doctors have further looked into what type of problems children face because of lack of sleep. According to a study completed at Northwestern University Medical Center, researchers found that children often have behavioral problems when they don't get enough sleep. Without the right amount of sleep, children can acquire psychological disorders, such as anxiety and depression. Therefore, some factors that can cause sleep disorders are also factors that children face when they don't get enough sleep.

I have already discussed what sleep disorders can do to your child in chapter 2. Now I am going to focus on why and how these sleep disorders develop. I will also look at how you can limit your child's chances of developing a sleep disorder and suggest solutions you can try if your child develops a sleeping disorder.

A child can develop a sleep disorder at almost any age. While most newborns don't tend to develop sleep disorders, it's not unheard of. However, most sleep disorders start around the age of four to six months, especially when the baby's brain becomes more active. For example, your child can have a nightmare about a birthday party coming up, even their own, if they feel you are anxious about it or talk about it often. This is one reason why many pediatricians and child psychologists tell parents they need to talk in a calm and soothing voice as much as possible around their baby or toddler. The truth is, adults never know how their young child is going to interpret the situation, and especially for babies and toddlers, this interpretation heavily depends on how they hear their parents talk about a subject. If your child senses anger in your voice, they are going to believe you are angry over the subject, such as their birthday party, even if you are just frustrated because the bakery screwed up on the cake.

Another reason that can make a child's imagination run wild is not getting a nap during the day. Unfortunately, this can happen to any parent and any child. No matter how hard you try, the doctor might schedule a visit during naptime, or you might have a family emergency you need to attend to. In other words, you won't always be able to follow the schedule that you have set for your child, which can make your child's brain become more active once they are able to get sleep. This happens because your child becomes overtired because of missing their nap, which causes their brain to become overactive. This, in return, can cause nightmares or a night terror.

How to Prevent Sleep Disorders

In reality, sometimes there is no way to prevent a sleep disorder. A child naturally has an immature nervous system, which can cause them to wet the bed. Furthermore, a child cannot control if their throat is going to be big enough for the tonsils and adenoids when they sleep. This is just a part that he is born with. A child has a naturally active imagination, which can create such things as nightmares and night terrors. However, this doesn't mean that you shouldn't try to find an underlying factor. For example, if you just moved into a new community, your child might have trouble falling asleep because it is a new location. This is typical with a baby or toddler but also an underlying factor. You know that your child is having sleep onset problems because of their new environment, and once they get used to it, they will be able to sleep better. Of course, keeping up with your child's naptime and bedtime routine and explaining that this is their new home will help your child adjust.

One way to prevent any onset of sleeping problems, which can develop into sleeping disorders, is to remember to remain as calm as possible when there is a struggle with your child or in the environment that your child is in. A baby can easily sense when something is not right with their parents. They know when their parents are angry, happy, sad, or frustrated. A baby is also very empathic once they can sense a negative emotion. They can feel this way, which can cause them to become fussy and cry. This can upset them for bedtime, which can cause them to take longer and need more comfort as they fall asleep.

Taking care of your child's needs is another way to prevent sleep disorders. A child, whether a baby or toddler, understands when their needs are met and when they are not met. When needs are not being met, this can cause an internal struggle with your child. For example, they can feel that you are not giving them what they need, which can make them uncomfortable and untrusting of you. This can quickly create insomnia or another type of sleep disorder because your baby is not completely happy. Unfortunately, it isn't always easy to understand directly what your child needs at the moment. This is especially true for new parents as they are just learning how to care for a child. When this happens, it is important to remember that as long as you keep trying, remain calm, and do what you can to find out what your child needs, you will be able to gain their trust and help them through any sleeping problems or disorders they could be acquiring.

It is important to remember that every parent makes mistakes and stumbles every now and then. There are no perfect parents, no matter how hard they try. The trick is to learn from your mistakes, gain experience, and give your child unconditional love and care. With this mindset, you will be able to accomplish your parenting goals, and your child will continue to thrive in a wonderful and loving home.

Chapter 14

What Is Sleep Paralysis?

Usually associated with narcolepsy, sleep paralysis is more serious. It affects 20% to 40% of the people in the US and it begins at the age of 10. Episodes decrease once a person reaches the age of 17 years old. It occurs when you wake up from your sleep or when you fall asleep. This sleep disorder makes you unable to move muscles, limbs or your whole body. It usually lasts for ten seconds to a couple of minutes and is sometimes accompanied by hallucinations. Such hallucinations are auditory, tactile or visual in nature.

Medical experts say sleep paralysis may be genetic. Other things that cause it include:

1. Sleeplessness

2. Drug use

3. Lying on the back

4. Changing schedules

5. Medical or mental conditions

In treating sleep paralysis, you need to tell your body to be ready to get proper sleep. You have to eat properly during the day because the kind of nutrients you receive will have an effect on the kind of sleep you will have. Get at least six to eight hours of sleep and refrain from napping often so that you will not experience sleep paralysis frequently.

At night, sleep on your side because lying on the back has been proven to promote sleep paralysis episodes. If you are having an attack, do not focus on trying to wake up. Instead, remove them from your mind as this should decrease the onset of these episodes.

Visit your physician if you continuously experience sleep paralysis. You may be having another health issue which needs to be addressed in order that your sleep paralysis doesn't occur again.

Doctors usually give two medications for sleep paralysis and one of them is Ritalin. This must be taken each morning for it to work throughout the day. This medication regulates sleep cycles and treats sleep paralysis experienced by some adults.

Another medication is Clonazepam to be taken prior to sleeping. It also regulates sleep patterns, but in a different way from Ritalin. It is said to be more effective than Ritalin in treating sleep paralysis.

Always visit your doctor for a follow-up checkup so that he will know if the medicine prescribed for you worked or not. He will also check to see if the sleep paralysis attacks you are suffering are decreasing or not.

Chapter 15

Understanding Nocturia As A Common Sleeping Disorder

Another sleep disorder is nocturia and it is the urge to go to the bathroom and excessively urinate during sleeping hours. It can be irritating for sufferers because they wake up every now and then just to urinate. This leaves them lacking a restful sleep. There are different causes of nocturia. This disorder has both treatable and untreatable stubborn symptoms.

To treat nocturia, you have to first undergo behavioral changes. You may have to limit your fluid intake after a particular hour. You may also need to elevate your legs during bedtime and take naps during the day. You may also have to wear compression hosiery to improve the flow of blood to your legs and lower the possibility of fluid buildup.

There are medications that doctors prescribe for nocturia. Furosemide or Bumetanide helps control the production of urine at night. Another prescription which stops or slows down bladder spasms is Darifenacin. Doctors also prescribe Desmopressin, a drug that mimics hormones that make the kidneys release less urine.

A medication that blocks receptors on the wall of the bladder which leads to an excessively active bladder is trospium chloride. A drug that lessens urine produced is Imipramine while Tolterodine, Oxybutynin and Solifenacin relax bladder muscles which reduces nighttime urination.

The Chinese use a holistic alternative treatment such as acupuncture to treat nocturia. This treatment concentrates on the kidneys so as to decrease urine produced and takes away liver problems leading to urinary imbalance. It also focuses on bladder, tummy, kidney and spleen imbalances.

There are also Chinese herbs that treat nocturia such as Psoralea, Ootheca Mantidis and Chinese Dodder Seeds. These herbs concentrate on healing the kidneys. Chinese Foxglove Root and Dried Cinnamon Bark are the herbs that nourish the kidneys. Astragalus root helps toughen the spleen so the urge to urinate frequently is controlled.

Chapter 16

An Overview Of Sleep Talking

It is medically referred to as somniloquy, but in layman's term it is known as sleep talking. It is temporary and harmless and has no effect on sleep, but when you suffer from it, it can be irritating to people who sleep with you.

When one talks in his sleep, he speaks briefly or gives out simple sounds. There are times that the sufferer makes long speeches. The sufferer will not remember what was said. Sleep talking is sometimes caused by other sleep problems, emotional stress, fever and various external factors.

When you have sleep talking episodes, you may utter random words, complete sentences or even vulgar phrases. This is because your brain is relaxed during sleep. There are rare cases when people yell and this awakens others around you.

Children are the ones usually affected by sleep talking. Statistics say 50% of children from the age group 3-10 years have conversations while sleeping. Ten percent talk as they sleep more than once per week. Approximately 5% of adults talk while sleeping.

There is an aggressive kind of somniloquy and this is RBD which was explained previously. This kind of sleep disorder has violent episodes where the sufferer shouts, screams and kicks. He doesn't remember what he did and is usually surprised when he hears of such an episode. RBD happens due to anxiety, illness, brain disorders and extreme stress.

One of the ways to treat sleep talking is to get a sufficient amount of sleep. Medical experts say this disorder happens to people who suffer from sleep deprivation. If they rest regularly, then this will lessen episodes of sleep talking.

It is important to lower stress in your daily life in order to stop talking in your sleep. Stress is one factor that increases its severity and frequency. Stay away from stressors and do stress-relieving activities such as having an aromatherapy massage, doing yoga or meditating.

You also have to stay away from alcohol before bedtime because this can worsen sleep talking and interrupt your sleep patterns. Before sleeping, do not consume large meals nor should you eat late-night snacks as these also disrupt sleep. It is important not to consume food less than 4 hours prior to sleeping. It's also a good idea to stay away from coffee or sugary foods.

If talking in your sleep disturbs your partner or if you think that your sleep talking is a side effect of yet another sleep disorder, then you should pay your doctor a visit. He will be able to diagnose your problem and give you an in-depth treatment program.

Chapter 17

How To Deal With Snoring?

Snoring occurs if your breathing patterns when sleeping create noise. This sleep disorder happens to all genders and ages and according to statistics, it affects around 90 million adults in America. Usually, it affects men and those who are overweight. Statistics say 45% of adults occasionally snore while 25% snore habitually.

Occasional snoring is not really serious, but it disturbs the person lying next to the snorer. Habitual snoring is considered serious because it also disturbs the sleeping pattern of the snorer. This sleep problem results in sleep that is not relaxing and leads to sleepiness and tiredness during the daytime.

One method of curing or reducing snoring is to lose weight. Once you have lost weight, the fatty tissue in your airway will be reduced, making oxygen flow more smoothly.

Another way to lessen snoring is to sleep on your side. Insert a small ball in your sleepwear since this will prevent you from rolling on your back as you sleep.

For your neck not to bend, sleep without using a pillow. Raise the head of your bed so that breathing will become easier.

Smoking irritates the membranes found in your nose and throat and they block your airways. Avoid people who smoke because secondhand smoke is also a contributing factor.

Do not consume alcohol or snacks three hours prior to sleeping at night. Try to avoid milky products prior to going to bed because they generate mucus in your throat.

Stay away from sleeping pills or antihistamines as they relax your throat muscles and obstruct breathing.

You can also buy products that will help you cure snoring. These include snore pillows and nasal strips and sprays.

If your snoring gets worse and causes a strain in your relationship, then you need to see your doctor. You may have to use medical devices such as dental appliances, continuous pressure machines, lower-jaw positioners, oral devices, implants and tongue-retaining devices. In extreme cases, the adenoids and tonsils are removed.

Conclusion

Sleep advances sleep, and it is a false notion to believe that if you keep a baby awake throughout the day, they will sleep better at night. The turnaround is, in reality, apparent.

In these early weeks, a baby is truly versatile and can, for the most part, sleep in any room. It is essential to look for their tired signs and foresee that they will happen. At this early age, tired symptoms start around 1 - 1 ½ hour after they wake.

A newborn will, as a rule, wake themselves with appetite, hence nurse them straight away. You can generally change their diaper halfway through the feed. This will wake them up if they are falling asleep to ensure they complete a full feed.

A few babies during their initial two weeks are sleepy day and night. If you have a sleepy baby during the day, ensure that you wake them for a feed like clockwork. This will enable them to build up their day/night rhythm just as giving them the required supplements for development.

Babies love to suck; in this manner, a pacifier can come in handy. If your baby stirs and wakes after just 20 minutes of sleep, utilize the pacifier to encourage them to return to sleep for another cycle. Be sure not to use it if they are expected for a feed.

If you believe you have tried everything to enable your baby to settle and sleep, and nothing is by all accounts working; they are not satisfied and content, and you are depleted, at that point the time has come to look for individual expert assistance. Your baby depends on you to function well and not be consumed from the absence of sleep. By getting expert assistance early; analysis can be made, and sleep can be recovered inside two or three days and will enable your baby to sleep well.

CPSIA information can be obtained
at www.ICGtesting.com
Printed in the USA
BVHW091507150221
600148BV00002B/11